W9-AHF-150

Essentials of dental caries

Essentials of dental caries

The disease and its management

Third edition

Edwina Kidd

Emeritus Professor of Cariology
Guy's, King's and St Thomas' Dental Institute
King's College
University of London

OXFORD
UNIVERSITY PRESS

OXFORD
UNIVERSITY PRESS

Great Clarendon Street, Oxford OX2 6DP

Oxford University Press is a department of the University of Oxford.
It furthers the University's objective of excellence in research, scholarship,
and education by publishing worldwide in

Oxford New York

Auckland Cape Town Dar es Salaam Hong Kong Karachi
Kuala Lumpur Madrid Melbourne Mexico City Nairobi
New Delhi Shanghai Taipei Toronto

With offices in

Argentina Austria Brazil Chile Czech Republic France Greece
Guatemala Hungary Italy Japan South Korea Poland Portugal
Singapore Switzerland Thailand Turkey Ukraine Vietnam

Oxford is a registered trade mark of Oxford University Press
in the UK and in certain other countries

Published in the United States
by Oxford University Press Inc., New York

Database right Oxford University Press (maker)
First edition published by IOP Publishing Limited 1987
Second edition published by Oxford University Press 1997
This edition published 2005

A catalogue record for this title is available from the British Library

Library of Congress Cataloguing in Publication Data

Kidd, Edwina A. M.
Essentials of dental caries / Edwina Kidd.–3rd ed.
Includes bibliographical references and index.
1. Dental caries.
[DNLM: 1. Dental Caries. WU 270 K47ea 2005] I. Title.
RK331.K43 2005   617,6'7–dc22   2004019794

ISBN 0 19 852978 3 (Pbk. : alk. paper)

10 9 8 7 6 5 4 3 2 1

Typeset by EXPO Holdings Sdn. Bhd., Malaysia
Printed in Italy
on acid-free paper by Grafiche Industriali

Preface

The first edition of this little book was published by John Wright in 1987, having been commissioned over a postprandial brandy at the George Inn, Southwark, London. The idea was to produce an easy-to-read, clinically relevant text for the junior undergraduate. The authors were frustrated by the complexity of the cariology texts available at that time which, they felt, lacked the clinical dimension which would take the biology to the chairside.

The book has also been used by dental nurses, dental health educators, hygienists, and therapists. In addition scientists working in the dental field have found this a useful introduction to clinical cariology. This title has now found its way all over the world and is produced in CD-ROM form for some universities.

The second, and now this third edition have been published by Oxford University Press. The aim is still to produce a simple text to serve as a springboard for further study. This books seeks to complement more comprehensive texts which are referenced. Other references include relevant systematic reviews, review articles, and some original papers. The latter must be regarded as the idiosyncratic choice of the author, but this does not devalue them in any way.

E.A.M. KIDD

London
August 2004

Acknowledgements

The manuscript was word processed by Miss Audrey Fernandes, and I am grateful for her patience and care.

This edition has a single author (EAMK) because Sally Joyston-Bechal is now retired. However, Sally has criticized this new edition. Her logic and attention to detail, as well as to deadlines, are irreplaceable.

E.A.M. KIDD

Contents

CHAPTER 9: THE OPERATIVE MANAGEMENT OF CARIES

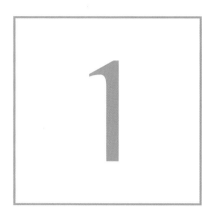

Introduction

1.1 WHAT IS CARIES?

Dental caries is a process that may take place on any tooth surface in the oral cavity where dental plaque is allowed to develop over a period of time.

Plaque formation is a natural, physiological process which will be described in more detail in the next section. Plaque is an example of a **biofilm**, which means it is not a haphazard collection of bacteria but a community of microorganisms attached to a surface. This community works together, having a collective physiology. The bacteria in the biofilm are always metabolically active. Some of the bacteria are capable of fermenting a suitable dietary carbohydrate substrate (such as the sugars sucrose and glucose), to produce acid, causing the plaque pH to fall to below 5 within 1–3 minutes. Repeated falls in pH may in time result in **demineralization** of the tooth surface. However, the acid produced is neutralized by saliva, so the pH increases and mineral may be regained. This is called **remineralization**. The cumulative results of the de- and remineralization processes may be a net loss of mineral and a carious lesion that can be seen. Alternatively, the changes may be so slight that a carious lesion never becomes apparent (Figure 1.1).[1]

From this description it becomes obvious that the carious process is an ubiquitous, natural process. The formation of the biofilm and its metabolic activity cannot be prevented, but disease progression can be controlled so that a clinically visible lesion never forms: alternatively, the process can be arrested and even advanced carious lesions may become inactive. However, the other side of the coin is that progression of the lesion into dentine can ultimately result in bacterial invasion and death of the pulp and spread of infection into the periapical tissues, causing pain.

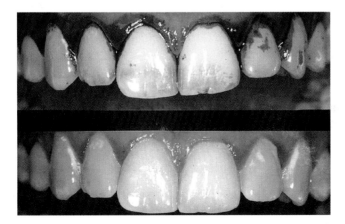

Figure 1.1. The upper anterior teeth of a young adult. In the upper picture, a disclosing agent reveals the plaque, while in the lower picture the plaque has been removed. White spot lesions are visible on the canines, but not on other tooth surfaces, although plaque is present.

1.2   THE CARIOUS PROCESS AND THE CARIOUS LESION

It is probably unfortunate that the word 'caries' is used to denote both the carious process and the carious lesion which forms as a result of that process. The process occurs in the biofilm at the tooth or cavity surface; the interaction of the biofilm with the dental tissues results in the lesion in the tooth. The metabolic activity in the biofilm cannot be seen, but the lesion, which is its reflection or consequence, can be seen. Thus the dentist is working on a reflection, and there is a danger that the dentist might forget that the 'action' is in the biofilm.

Please stand in front of a mirror and look at your reflection. Do you like what you see, or could it be improved by some makeup, a shave, a new haircut, new clothes? You are of course concentrating on the real you and it probably would not occur to you to pick up a brick and smash the mirror! But if you now go into the clinic you will see dentists filling holes in teeth, and in a way they are smashing the mirror unless they have **also** concentrated on teaching the patient to modify the metabolic activity in the biofilm.

1.3   DENTAL PLAQUE[2]

It is thought-provoking that the human body is composed of some 10^{14} cells, but only about 10% of these are mammalian; the remainder are resident microflora. Although a newborn baby's mouth is sterile, it soon acquires microbes, usually from the mother via saliva. More than 300 species of microorganisms have been identified in the mouth.

Dental plaque is an adherent deposit of bacteria and their products, which forms on all tooth surfaces and is the cause of caries. As already mentioned, plaque is a biofilm—a community of microorganisms attached to a surface. The populations of bacteria interact and the properties of the community are more than the sum of the constituent species. The organisms are organized into a three-dimensional structure enclosed in a matrix of extracellular material derived from the cells themselves and their environment.

Dental plaque formation can be described in sequential stages:
• Formation of **pellicle**: an acellular, proteinaceous film, derived from saliva, which forms on a 'naked' tooth surface.
• Within 0–4 hours, single bacterial cells colonize the pellicle. A large proportion of these are streptococci *(S. sanguis, S. oralis, S. mitis)*. There are also *Acintomyces* species and Gram-negative bacteria. Only about 2% of the initial streptococci are mutans streptococci, and this is of interest because these organisms are particularly associated with the initiation of the carious process.
• Over the next 4–24 hours the attached bacteria grow, leading to the formation of distinct **microcolonies**.
• In 1–14 days the **Streptococcus**-dominated plaque changes to a plaque dominated by **Actinomyces**. Thus the population shifts; this is called

microbial succession. The bacterial species become more diverse and the microcolonies continue to grow.
- In 2 weeks the plaque is mature but there are considerable site-to-site variations in its composition. Each site can be considered as unique and these local variations may explain why lesions progress in some sites but not others in the same mouth.

1.3.1 Pathogenic properties of cariogenic bacteria

There are a number of organisms, normally present in plaque, which can cause caries. These cariogenic bacteria can:
- transport sugars and convert them to acid (**acidogenic**)
- produce extracellular and intracellular polysaccharides which contribute to the plaque matrix; intracellular polysaccharides can be used for energy production and converted to acid when sugars are not available
- thrive at low pH (**aciduric**).

1.3.2 Which plaque bacteria cause caries?

There are a number of possibilities, each of which has consequences:
- The **specific plaque hypothesis** proposed that only a few organisms out of the diverse collection in the plaque flora were actively involved in the disease. Preventive measures targeting specific bacteria (e.g. immunization) would be a logical consequence of this hypothesis.
- The **non-specific plaque hypothesis** considered the carious process to be caused by the overall activity of the total plaque microflora. A consequence of this approach is that all plaque should be disturbed by mechanical plaque control (toothbrushing).
- The **ecological plaque hypothesis** proposes that the organisms associated with disease may be present at sound sites. Demineralization will result from a shift in the balance of these resident microflora driven by a change in the local environment. Frequent sugar intake (or decreased sugar clearance if salivary secretion is low) encourages the growth of acidogenic and aciduric species, thus predisposing a site to caries. The consequence of this hypothesis is that both mechanical cleaning and some restriction of sugar intake are important in controlling caries progression.

1.3.3 Where does caries occur?

Bacterial plaque is the essential precusor of caries and for this reason sites on the tooth surface which encourage plaque retention and stagnation are particularly prone to progression of lesions. These sites are:
- enamel in pits and fissures on occlusal surfaces of molars and premolars (Figure 1.2), buccal pits of molars, and palatal pits of maxillary incisors
- approximal enamel smooth surfaces just cervical to the contact point (Figure 1.3)

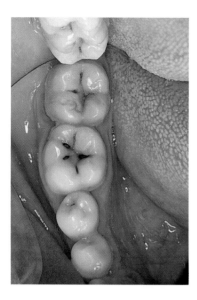

Figure 1.2. Occlusal caries in molars showing stained fissures. Cavities were present.

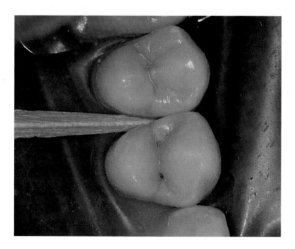

Figure 1.3. A carious lesion is present on the distal aspect of the upper first premolar. The lesion is shining up through the marginal ridge which shows a pinkish-grey discolouration.

- the enamel of the cervical margin of the tooth just coronal to the gingival margin (Figure 1.4a–c)
- in patients where periodontal disease has resulted in gingival recession, the area of plaque stagnation is on the exposed root surface (Figure 1.5)
- the margins of restorations, particularly those that are deficient or overhanging
- tooth surfaces adjacent to dentures (Figure 1.5) and bridges which make cleaning more difficult, thus encouraging plaque stagnation.

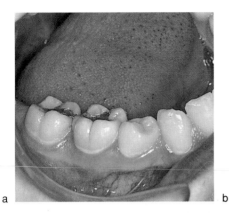
a

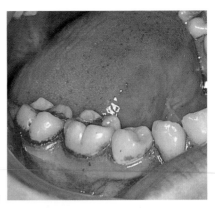
b

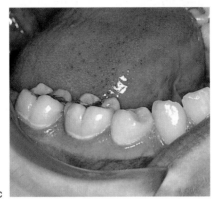
c

Figure 1.4. Caries of the enamel at the cervical margin of the lower molars: (a) The white spot lesions covered with plaque. (b) A red dye has been used to stain the plaque so that the patient can see the plaque clearly. (c) The patient has now removed the stained plaque with a toothbrush: the white spot lesions are now very obvious. Note they have formed in an area of plaque stagnation and this can been shown to the patient to demonstrate the importance of plaque removal.

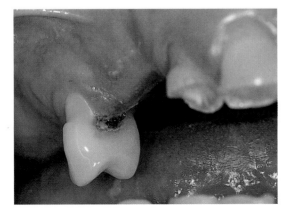

Figure 1.5. Caries on the exposed root surface of the mesial aspect of the upper premolar. Note the lesion is in an area of plaque stagnation adjacent to a removable denture. Dentine is also exposed buccally, but this has been cleaned and abraded by the toothbrush and is caries-free.

1.3.4 Is dental caries an infectious, preventable, disease?

No, perhaps it is neither. Although it is caused by bacteria, these are commensal organisms, not extraneous infecting invaders. The carious process cannot be prevented, because the activity in the biofilm is an ubiquitous, natural process. However, the progression of lesions can be controlled. These statements are contentious and may provoke strong reaction and interesting discussion from your teachers!

1.4 THE ROLE OF DIETARY CARBOHYDRATE

It is necessary for fermentable carbohydrates and plaque to be present on the tooth surface for a minimum length of time for acid to form and cause demineralization of dental enamel. These carbohydrates provide the plaque bacteria with the substrate for acid production and the synthesis of extracelluar polysaccharides. However, carbohydrates are not all equally cariogenic. Complex carbohydrates such as starch are relatively harmless because they are not completely digested in the mouth, but carbohydrates of low molecular weight (sugars) diffuse readily into plaque and are metabolized quickly by the bacteria. Thus, many sugar-containing foods and drinks cause a rapid drop in plaque pH to a level which can cause demineralization of dental enamel. The plaque remains acid for some time, taking 30–60 minutes to return to its normal pH (in the region of 7). The gradual return of pH to baseline values is a result of acids diffusing out of the plaque and buffers in the plaque and salivary film overlying it, exerting a neutralizing effect. Repeated and frequent consumption of sugar will keep plaque pH depressed and cause demineralization of the teeth.

The change in plaque pH may be represented graphically over a period of time following a glucose rinse (Figure 1.6). Such a graph is called a 'Stephan

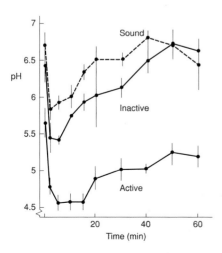

Figure 1.6. Stephan response curves obtained from sound occlusal surfaces, inactive occlusal carious lesions and deep, active occlusal carious cavities following a sucrose rinse in a group of 14-year-olds. Bars indicate standard errors.[3] (Reproduced by kind permission of Professor Fejerskov).

curve' after the person who first described it in 1944. Once a cavity, or hole, forms in the tooth, the plaque within it becomes even more efficient at producing acid. Lower pH values are recorded in plaque within cavities than in plaque on inactive lesions or sound surfaces in the same individuals.[3]

The synthesis of extracellular polysaccharides from sucrose is more rapid than from glucose, fructose, or lactose. Consequently, sucrose is the most cariogenic sugar, although the other sugars are also harmful. Since sucrose is also the sugar most commonly eaten, it is a very important cause of dental caries.

1.5 ENVIRONMENT OF THE TOOTH: SALIVA AND FLUORIDE

Under normal conditions the tooth is continually bathed in saliva. Saliva is supersaturated with calcium and phosphate ions and capable of remineralizing the very early stages of lesion formation, particularly when the fluoride ion is present. Fluoride slows down the progression of lesions.

When salivary flow is diminished or absent, there is increased food retention. Since salivary buffering capacity has been lost, an acid environment is encouraged and persists longer. This in turn encourages aciduric bacteria which relish the acid conditions and continue to metabolize carbohydrate in the low-pH environment. The stage is set for uncontrolled carious attack.

1.6 CLASSIFICATION OF DENTAL CARIES

Carious lesions can be classified in different ways; this section introduces and defines this terminology.

Lesions can be classified according to their anatomical site. Thus lesions may be found in **pits and fissures** or on **smooth surfaces**. Lesions may start on enamel (**enamel caries**) or on exposed root cementum and dentine (**root caries**).

Primary caries denotes lesions on unrestored surfaces. Lesions developing adjacent to fillings are referred to as either **recurrent or secondary caries**. **Residual caries** is demineralized tissue left in place before a filling is placed.

Carious lesions may also be classified according to their activity. A progressive lesion is described as an **active carious lesion** (Figure 1.1) whereas a lesion that may have formed earlier and then stopped is referred to as an **arrested** or **inactive carious lesion** (Figure 1.7, 1.8). This concept of activity is very important as it impinges directly on management because active lesions require active management. However, the distinction between active and arrested may not be straightforward. There will be a continuum of

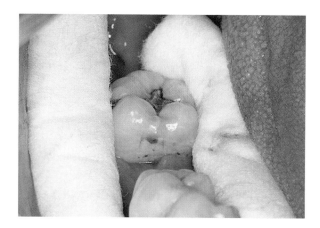

Figure 1.7. Arrested caries on the mesial aspect of the lower second molar. The lesion probably stopped progressing after extraction of the lower first molar.

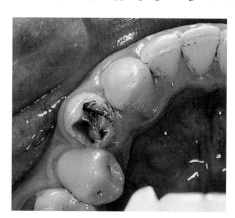

Figure 1.8. An arrested carious lesion in the lower first premolar. The lesion was well into dentine, but the tissue was hard and shiny. Note it is plaque-free. The tooth had been in this state for at least 10 years.

changes between active and arrested, and part of a lesion may be active while another part is arrested. This concept is totally logical because the lesion merely reflects the ecological balance in the overlying biofilm.

Different teeth and surfaces are involved, depending on the area of plaque stagnation and the severity of the carious challenge. Thus, with a very mild challenge only the most vulnerable teeth and surfaces are attacked, such as the cervical margin of the teeth or the occlusal pits and fissures of permanent molars. A moderate challenge may also involve the approximal surfaces of posterior teeth. A severe challenge will cause the anterior teeth, which normally remain caries-free, also to become carious.

Rampant caries is the name given to multiple active carious lesions occurring in the same patient, frequently involving surfaces of teeth that are usually caries-free. It may be seen in the permanent dentition of teenagers and is usually due to poor oral hygiene and taking frequent cariogenic snacks and sweet drinks between meals (Figure 1.9a–c). It is also seen in mouths

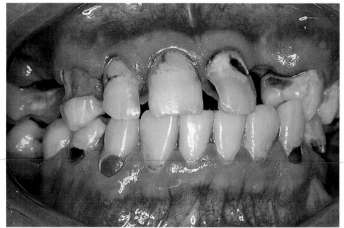

a

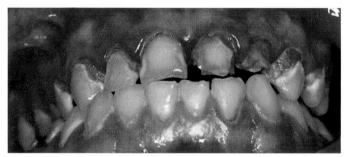

b

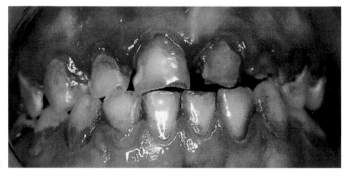

c

Figure 1.9. Rampant caries in young men: (a) Note these teeth look clean. This patient is now making strenuous attempts to remove plaque with a toothbrush. These lesions are on their way to arrest. Compare this with Figure 1.8.
(b) Despite help with oral hygiene, this patient is not keeping these teeth clean.
(c) The teeth are now disclosed and the plaque deposits are obvious. In addition, all this man's drinks are fizzy and sweet. This shows the devastating result of a combination of poor oral hygiene and a high-sugar diet.

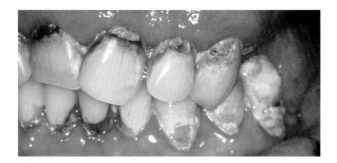

Figure 1.10. Radiation caries. This patient has been irradiated in the region of the salivary glands for the treatment of a malignant tumour. Heavy plaque deposits are obvious over the lesions.

where there is a sudden marked reduction in salivary flow (hyposalivation) (Figure 1.10). Radiation in the region of the salivary glands, used in the treatment of malignant tumours, is the most common cause of an acute reduction in salivary flow.

Early childhood caries is a term used to describe dental caries presenting in the primary dentition of young children.

Bottle caries or nursing caries are names used to describe a particular form of rampant caries in the primary dentition of infants and young children. The problem is found in an infant or toddler who falls asleep sucking a bottle (called a nursing bottle) which has been filled with sweetened fluids (including milk). Alternatively, nursing caries may be found in infants using a pacifier dipped in sweetener or in children who have a prolonged demand breast-feeding habit. The frequency of sugar intake combined with a low salivary flow at night are important in the development of this form of rampant caries. The clinical pattern is characteristic, with the four maxillary deciduous incisors most severely affected (Figure 1.11).

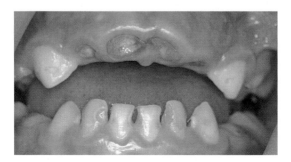

Figure 1.11. Rampant caries of deciduous teeth. The child continually sucked a dummy filled with rosehip syrup.

1.7 EPIDEMIOLOGY OF DENTAL CARIES

Epidemiology is the study of health and disease states in populations rather than individuals. The epidemiologist defines the frequency and severity of health problems in relation to such factors as age, sex, geography, race, economic status, nutrition, and diet. It is a bird's-eye view of a problem which attempts to delineate its magnitude, study its cause, and assess the efficacy of preventive and management strategies. Epidemiological surveys are of great importance to politicians because they should indicate areas of need where public money may be spent appropriately.

1.7.1 Measuring caries activity

Epidemiologists are interested in both the prevalence and the incidence of a disease. **Prevalence** is the proportion of a population affected by a disease or condition at a particular time. **Incidence** is a measurement of the rate at which a disease progresses. In order to measure incidence, therefore, two examinations are required—one at the beginning and one at the end of a given time period. The incidence of the condition is then the increase or decrease in the number of new cases occurring in a population within that time period.

Before incidence and prevalence can be recorded, a quantitative measurement is required that will reflect accurately the extent of the disease in a population. In the case of dental caries, the measurements of disease that are used are:

- the number of decayed teeth with untreated carious lesions (D)
- the number of teeth which have been extracted and are therefore missing (M)
- the number of filled teeth (F).

This measurement is known as the **DMF index** and is an arithmetic index of the cumulative caries attack in a population. DMF(T) is used to denote decayed, missing, and filled teeth; DMF(S) denotes decayed, missing, and filled surfaces in permanent teeth and therefore takes into account the number of surfaces attacked on each tooth. The similar indices for the primary dentition are def(t) and def(s) where e denotes extracted teeth (to differentiate from loss due to natural exfoliation) and f denotes filled teeth or surfaces.

1.7.2 Practical problems with DMF and def indices

There are some potential problems in the use of these indices. In young children missing deciduous teeth may have been lost as a result of natural exfoliation, and these must be differentiated from teeth lost due to caries. Permanent teeth are lost for reasons other than caries, such as trauma, extraction for orthodontic purposes and periodontal disease, or to facilitate the construction of dentures. For this reason missing teeth may be omitted from the indices and only decayed and filled surfaces included.

Epidemiologists take enormous trouble to achieve standardization of examination and recording techniques. They will practice and check their diagnoses during a clinical trial to try to ensure reproducibility. Despite this, even a trained and experienced worker will not be completely consistent on the same day, let alone consistent with others in studies spanning years.

In many populations there is a large filled component to the indices, and the dentists who have done the fillings are not standardized in their diagnosis of disease. Dentists do not practice and check their diagnostic reproducibility in the same way as epidemiologists. In addition, there is likely to be variation between dentists in their recording of disease. Epidemiologists carrying out national surveys may be limited in their access to clinical facilities because these surveys are not necessarily carried out in a dental surgery. Thus, access to good lighting, the ability to clean and dry teeth and the opportunity to examine radiographs may not be available. Unless radiographs are required for clinical care, it would be unethical to use ionizing radiation.

1.7.3 The relevance of diagnostic thresholds[4]

The recording of caries in epidemiological surveys is usually carried out at the 'caries into dentine' level of diagnosis. Enamel lesions are not recorded, which means that epidemiological surveys inevitably underestimate the caries problem. This may be very important because the earlier stages of lesion formation, which are not recorded, should be managed by non-operative preventive treatments so that the progression of lesions is controlled. The later stages (cavities) may also require restorations, in addition to preventive treatments. However, if only these are recorded, and those without cavities are described as 'caries-free', the politicians who commission the surveys in the first place may get a false impression of the dental care needed by the population.

This has indeed happened. In the early 1990s politicians (including dental politicians) in some developed countries gained the impression that because many children were described as 'caries-free', there was a danger of over-producing dentists. As a consequence of this unfortunate terminology and a lack of understanding of the carious process, some dental schools closed. However, it is now realized that in many people the carious process is delayed and thus lesions may present as cavities as the person grows older. In addition, the improvement in the caries status means there will be fewer extractions and thus many more teeth requiring dental care. For these reasons, more dental personnel are now needed. It must also be remembered that the arithmetic means of DMF(T) are meaningless at the level of the individual patient.

1.7.4 Caries prevalence[5]

Dental caries is ubiquitous in modern humans, and is the main cause of tooth loss in people of all ages. For most of the twentieth century caries was seen as a disease of economically developed countries, with a low prevalence in the developing world. By the late twentieth century this pattern was changing in two ways:

- There was evidence of a rise in caries experience in some developing countries. To give an example, studies in the 1990s show dental caries as a major problem in the former socialist countries of eastern Europe. These countries can be considered 'developing' in the economic sense, and the use of fluoride toothpastes and toothbrushes there is still low.
- By the late 1970s a marked reduction in caries experience among children and young adults was obvious in developed countries (Figure 1.12) although in 1983 there were considerable differences between countries.[6]

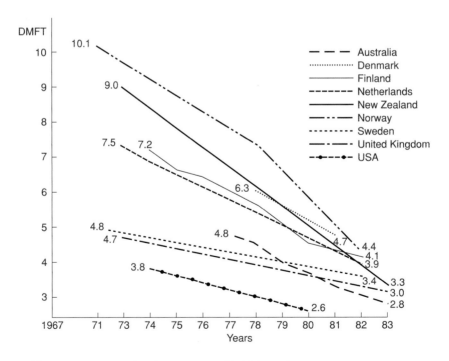

Figure 1.12, DMFT data from 12-year-old children of many countries demonstrating a decline in caries prevalence between 1967 and 1983. Note the considerable inter-country differences (data from the *WHO Global Oral Data Bank* (Renson *et al.*, 1986)[6]

The reasons for the decline in caries prevalence are not entirely under-stood, but experts consider the regular use of fluoridated toothpastes, prefer-ably twice a day, to be the most important single factor.[7]

Data from studies indicate that the decline in caries took various courses. For instance, in Norway it appears the decline started several years before the widespread use of fluoride toothpaste. In the Netherlands, water fluorida-tion, beginning in 1953, led to a reduction in caries prevalence but the decline soon became independent of water fluoridation, which was dis-continued in 1973.[8]

1.7.5 The position in the UK

Children

Figure 1.13 shows time trends in caries experience of children in England and Wales between 1973 and 1993. The end of the decline first became evident in the primary dentition (5-year-old data) with a levelling out becom-ing apparent in 12- and 14-year-old children in the early 1990s.[9]

Preliminary results of the 2003 Children's Dental Health in the UK survey have been released as this edition goes to press. There is little change between 1993 and 2003 in the obvious decay experience in 5-year-olds, but there has been a decrease in the average number of filled teeth in this age group. The picture for permanent teeth in older children is more positive with further reductions in obvious decay experience in 12- and 15-year-old children.

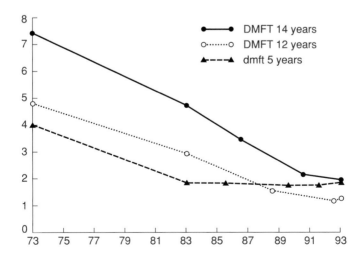

Figure 1.13. Time trends in caries experience of children in England and Wales between 1973 and 1993. (Reproduced by kind permission of the *International Dental Journal.*[9])

The reduction in caries experience has not occurred evenly across all tooth surfaces. As caries prevalence falls, the least susceptible sites (smooth and approximal surfaces) reduce by the greatest proportion, while the most susceptible sites (occlusal surfaces) reduce by the smallest proportion.

There are large regional inequalities in dental health, with people in Northern Ireland, Scotland and the north of England having the worst caries status (Figure 1.14).[10] In addition, caries is much worse in areas of social

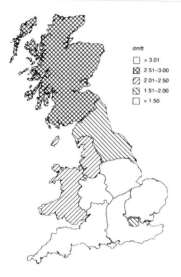

Figure 1.14. Dental caries experience (dmft) of 5-year-old children in Great Britain (BASCD coordinated National Health Service Dental Epidemiological Programme survey of 5-year-old children, 1999/2000). (Reproduced by kind permission of Blackwell Munksgaard).

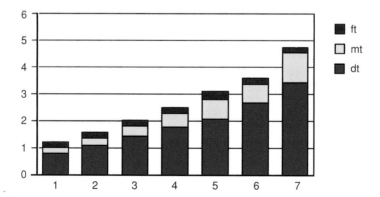

Figure 1.15. Mean number of decayed, missing and filled teeth by 'deprivation category' (DEPCAT score) in Scottish school children aged 5 years.[11] (Reproduced from Sweeney, P. C., Nugent, Z. L., and Pitts, N. B. (1999) Deprivation and dental caries status of 5-year-old children in Scotland. *Community Dent. Oral Epidemiol.* **27**, 152-9 by kind permission of Blackwell Munksgaard).

deprivation and Figure 1.15 shows the dmft levels for 5-year-old children in Scotland plotted against DEPCAT status (a measure of social deprivation based on postcodes).[11] A clear link between caries levels and DEPCAT scores, which reflect socio-economic conditions, is obvious. It can also be seen that many decayed teeth remain unfilled; presumably because many practitioners are unwilling to spend time restoring deciduous teeth.

Adults

National surveys of adult dental health, carried out in UK every 10 years, show steady and substantial improvements with the most dramatic improvements being in young adults. The bulk of filled teeth is now in older adults. Northern Ireland, Scotland and the north of England remain the parts of the UK with the poorest dental health.[12]

Older people

Caries is the commonest cause of tooth loss in all ages but edentulousness has decreased in UK adults. In 1968, 37% of the population over 16 had no teeth but by 1998 this had decreased to 13%. This means that people are coming dentate to old age, and caries in elderly people can be a particular problem because:

• oral hygiene may be poor if people are not able to brush or forget to do so
• salivary flow may be reduced by medications
• diet may change, with more sugar consumed.

The dental state of older people in residential homes is a disgrace. The clients are there because they can no longer look after themselves, and yet carers often do not clean mouths. It is unacceptable to ignore such an intimate part of the body—it eats, its speaks, it smiles, it kisses—and our profession must face this challenge (Figure 1.16).[13]

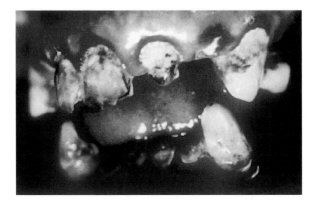

Figure 1.16. Gross caries in a client in a residential home. (Reproduced by kind permission of Dr Debra Simons).

1.8 MODIFYING THE CARIOUS PROCESS

Caries is a multifactorial disease. The cause is pH fluctuations in the bacterial plaque, but these in turn may be influenced by such factors oral hygiene, diet, fluoride and salivary flow. In addition a number of other variables are important such as social class, income, education, knowledge, attitudes and behaviour.

Figure 1.17 is a diagrammatic representation of the carious process. It makes the point that the process does not have to progress. When the destructive forces outweigh the reparative powers of saliva, the process will progress. Conversely, if the reparative forces outweigh the destructive forces, the process will arrest. Early diagnosis is important because, once carious lesions have cavitated, only operative intervention can replace the tissue. Fillings do not prevent caries, because new lesions can develop adjacent to restorations. If fillings are to last, preventive non-operative treatments must go hand-in-hand with operative treatment.

The basis of preventive, non-operative treatment is modification of one or more of the factors involved in the carious process. Since the process usually takes months or years to destroy the tooth, time is on the patient's side.

The dentist can help the patient modify the carious process in a number of ways:

- **Oral hygiene instruction.** Since the process is the metabolic activity in the biofilm, plaque removal using a fluoride toothpaste is very important (Chapter 4).

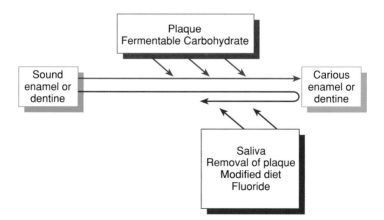

Figure 1.17. A diagrammatic representation of the carious process as an alternating process of destruction and repair. Sound enamel or dentine will become carious in time if plaque bacteria are given the substrate they need to produce acid. However, progression of lesions can be arrested by improving plaque control, modifying diet, and using fluoride appropriately.

- **Dietary advice.** Relatively simple measures, such as reducing the frequency of consumption of sugar and confining it to meal times, are usually sufficient (Chapter 5).
- **Appropriate use of fluoride.** Fluoride used in toothpaste, water, or mouthwashes and applied topically will delay progression of the lesion (Chapter 6).
- **Operative treatments.** Holes in teeth that are not cleansable are likely to progress. The role of operative dentistry in caries management is to facilitate plaque control (Chapter 9).

It is salutary to note that all the non-operative treatments require the patient's active cooperation. An important role for the dental profession, therefore, is to provide patients with knowledge so they understand their essential role in this control. In addition, patients need to be persuaded to accept responsibility for their own mouths (Chapter 8).

Further reading and references

1. Fejerskov, O. and Kidd, E. A. M. (eds) (2003) *Dental caries.* Ch.6: Caries diagnosis: 'a mental resting place on the way to intervention'? Blackwell Munksgaard, Oxford.
2. Fejerskov, O. and Kidd, E. A. M. (eds) (2003) *Dental caries.* Ch.3: The oral microflora and biofilms on teeth. Blackwell Munksgaard, Oxford.
3. Fejerskov, O., Scheie, A., and Manji, F. (1992) The effect of sucrose on plaque pH in the primary and permanent dentition of caries active and inactive Kenyan children. *J. Dent. Res.,* **71**, 25–31.
4. Fejerskov, O. and Kidd, E. A. M. (eds) (2003) *Dental caries.* Ch.9: Caries epidemiology, with special emphasis on diagnostic standards. Blackwell Munksgaard, Oxford.
5. Burt, B. A. and Eklund, S. A. (1999) *Dentistry, dental practice and the community.* Ch. 19: Dental caries. W B Saunders, Philadelphia.
6. Renson, C. E. (1986) Changing patterns of dental caries: a survey on 20 countries. *Ann. Acad. Med. Singapore,* **15**, 284–298.
7. Bratthal, D., Hänsel Petersson, G., and Sundberg, H. (1996) Reasons for the caries decline: What do the experts believe? *Eur. J. Oral. Sci.,* **104**, 416–422.
8. Marthaler, T. M. (2004) Changes in dental caries 1953–2003. *Caries Res.,* **38**, 173–181.
9. Downer, M. C. (1994) Caries prevalence in the UK. *Int. Dent J.,* **44**, 365–370.
10. British Association for the Study of Community Dentistry (BASCD). Epidemiology Programme (http://www.dundee.ac.uk/dhsru/bascd/bascd.htm).
11. Sweeney, P. C., Nugent, Z. L., and Pitts, N. B. (1999) Deprivation and dental caries status of 5-year-old children in Scotland. *Community Dent. Oral Epidemiol.,* **27**, 152–159.
12. Nuttall, N., Steele, J. G., Nunn, J., *et al.* (2001) *A Guide to the UK Adult Dental Health Survey 1998.* BDJ Books, London.
13. Simons, D., Kidd, E. A. M., and Beighton, D. (1999) Oral health of elderly occupants in residential homes. *Lancet,* **353**, 1761.

Clinical and histological features of carious lesions

2.1   INTRODUCTION

This chapter describes the clinical appearances of carious lesions on smooth, occlusal, and root surfaces and relates these appearances to their histological features. Enamel and dentine are considered together because:

- This is the way the clinician meets them.
- Changes in dentine during caries progression and arrest cannot be understood without considering spread of the enamel lesion.
- Dentine changes occur before the enamel lesion cavitates. Removal of the biofilm will arrest the lesion in dentine as well as the lesion in enamel. Remember, the lesion, in both enamel and dentine, entirely reflects the activity of the biofilm.

2.2   BASIC ENAMEL AND DENTINE STRUCTURE

Sound enamel consists of crystals of hydroxyapatite packed tightly together in an orderly arrangement (the enamel prisms). The crystals are so tightly packed that the enamel has a glass-like appearance and it is translucent, allowing the colour of the dentine to shine through it. Even though crystal packing is very tight, each crystal is actually separated from its neighbours by tiny intercrystalline spaces or pores. These spaces are filled with water and organic material. When enamel is exposed to acids produced in the microbial biofilm, mineral is removed from the surface of the crystal which shrinks in size. Thus, the intercrystalline spaces enlarge and the tissue becomes more porous. This increase in porosity can be seen clinically as a white spot.

Dentine is a vital tissue permeated by tubules containing the cell processes of the odontoblasts. This vital tissue defends itself from any assault, such as caries, by tubular sclerosis. This is the deposition of mineral along and within the dentinal tubules resulting in their gradual occlusion. In addition, the odontoblasts form tertiary dentine at the pulp–dentine border in response to the stimulus. Both these reactions are protective because they make the dentine less permeable.

2.3   THE FIRST VISIBLE SIGN OF CARIES ON AN ENAMEL SURFACE

The earliest visible sign of enamel caries is the 'white spot lesion'. To see the white spot lesion the plaque overlying it must be removed with a brush and the tooth thoroughly dried with a three-in-one syringe (Figure 1.1). This can be done occlusally (Figure 2.1) as well as buccally (Figure 2.2) or lingually. The active lesion is matt and feels rough if a sharp probe is gently drawn across it.

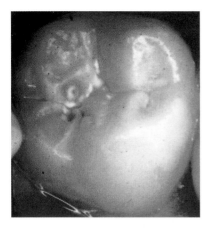

Figure 2.1. A white spot lesion at the entrance to the fissure on a molar.

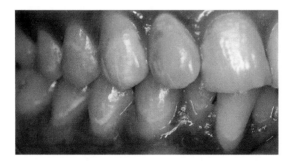

Figure 2.2. White spot lesions buccal to the lower premolars. These lesions are arrested. They are shiny, plaque-free, and remote from the gingival margin. The upper canine erupted slowly and was plaque covered for much of this time. A white spot lesion (now arrested) covers most of its labial face. The white spot lesions at the cervical margins of the upper incisors are plaque covered and may be active.

2.3.1 What is happening histologically?

A beautiful series of scanning electron microscope (SEM) studies, carried out in orthodontic patients due to have a premolar extracted, showed what was happening at the tooth surface. Bands allowing plaque to accumulate beneath them were put onto teeth. After 4 weeks they were removed and the classic matt, chalky white spots had formed. The SEM pictures showed that after 4 weeks of plaque accumulation there was marked dissolution of surface enamel (Figure 2.3). This partly explains why the surface is matt. Regular plaque control was now re-established and 3 weeks later the surface was hard and shiny and the white spot less obvious. Now the SEM pictures showed abrasion of the surface: the eroded area had been partly removed (Figure 2.4).

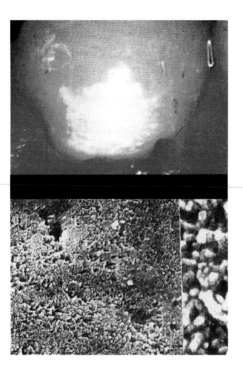

Figure 2.3. A clinical and SEM picture of a white spot lesion formed under an orthodontic band after 4 weeks of plaque stagnation. Clinically, the lesion is opaque with a matt surface. Ultrastructurally, there is dissolution of the perikymata overlappings and dissolution of the surface enamel. (Originally published in *Textbook of Clinical Cariology* (Munksgaard, 1994) and reproduced with permission.)

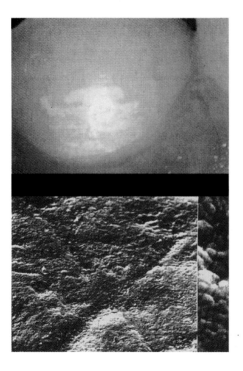

Figure 2.4. A clinical and SEM picture of a white spot lesion formed under an orthodontic band after renewal of plaque control. The lesion surface is now shiny and hard as a result of abrasion or polishing of the partly dissolved surface of the active lesion. (Originally published in *Textbook of Clinical Cariology* (Munksgaard, 1994) and reproduced with permission.)

2.3.2 Appearance of the white spot lesion in polarized light

In Figure 2.5 a white spot lesion on a smooth surface has been sectioned longitudinally. The section is in water and viewed in polarized light. The main part of the lesion (the **body** of the lesion) is seen as a dark area deep to a relatively well mineralized **surface zone**. The body of the lesion is porous and when the section is in water these pores have a volume in excess of 5%. The surface zone, on the other hand, is only about 1% demineralized.

If the section is now taken out of water and put into a liquid called quinoline, dark areas now outline the body of the lesion. These are called **dark zones** and have a pore volume of 2–4%. The areas look dark because there are big holes and little holes in the enamel and quinoline, being a big molecule, cannot get into the little holes which remain filled with air giving a dark

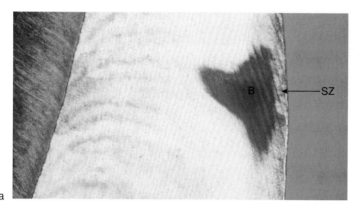

a

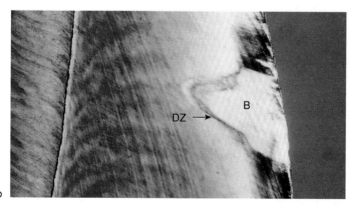

b

Figure 2.5. (a) Longitudinal ground section through a small lesion of enamel caries on a smooth surface examined in water with polarized light. The lesion is cone shaped. The body of the lesion (B) appears dark beneath a relatively intact surface zone (SZ). (b) The same section as in (a), now examined in quinoline with the polarizing microscope. A dark zone (DZ) can be seen outlining the lesion. The body (B) of the lesion appears translucent.

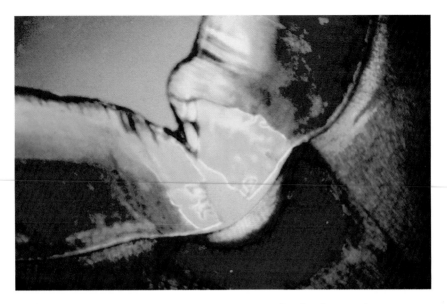

Figure 2.6. Longitudinal ground section of a natural occlusal carious lesion examined in quinoline in polarized light. The lesion forms in three directions, guided by prism direction assuming the shape of a cone with its base towards the enamel–dentine junction. The undermining shape of this lesion is purely a function of anatomy.

appearance. The body of the lesion, which looked dark in water, now looks translucent because quinoline has the same refractive index as enamel and has entered the porous spaces.

A section through a white spot lesion on an occlusal surface is seen in Figure 2.6. The occlusal lesion forms on the walls of the fissure in the area of plaque stagnation. This can been seen clinically on the sloping fissure walls at the fissure entrance (Figure 2.1). The dentine is involved in the lesion in Figure 2.6, but despite this, notice that the surface enamel is not yet cavitated.

2.3.3 Arrest of lesions

Inactive or arrested white spot lesions have a shiny surface and may be brown in colour, having picked up exogenous stains from the mouth (Figures 1.7 and 2.7). These lesions cannot be detected by gently drawing a sharp probe across them because they feel the same as normal enamel. Histologically these lesions show wide, well-developed dark zones at the front of the lesion within the body of the lesion and at the surface of the lesion (Figure 2.8).

It is very important to realize that the carious process can be arrested by simple clinical measures such as improved plaque control with a fluoride

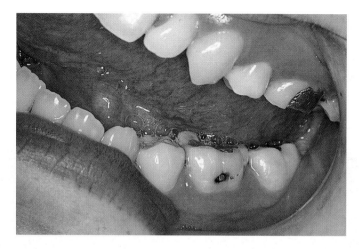

Figure 2.7. Arrested lesions on the buccal aspect of the lower first molar. A small amalgam restoration is also present. These lesions are likely to have formed years earlier at the gingival margin (compare with Figure 1.4, which shows an active lesion).

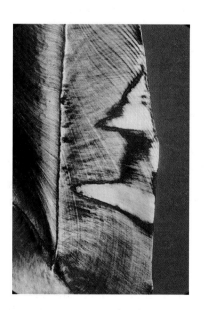

Figure 2.8. Longitudinal ground section of an arrested carious lesion in a tooth extracted from a patient aged 65 years. The section is examined in quinoline with polarized light and shows wide, well-developed dark zones at the advancing front of the lesion, within the body of the lesion and at the surface of the lesion.

toothpaste and altered diet. It is therefore the clinician's responsibility to detect enamel caries in its earliest form by careful visual inspection of teeth after cleaning and drying. The clinician can now help the patient tip the balance in favour of arrest rather than progression of lesions. An arrested white spot is more resistant to acid attack than sound enamel. It may be regarded as scar tissue and should not be attacked with a dental drill.

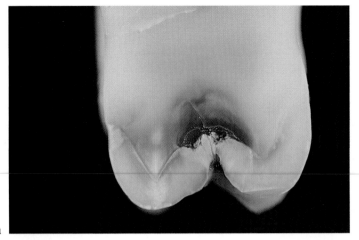

a

b

Figure 2.9. A sharp probe has been jammed into the white spot lesion on the buccal aspect of this extracted molar. (a) shows the lesion before probing and (b) shows the probe and the resulting damage. On the occlusal surface the enamel lesion has formed on the walls of the fissure and the lesion at the enamel–dentine junction is much under than the lesion the dentist can see at the enamel surface.

2.3.4 Clinical implications of subsurface porosity

Subsurface porous lesions can be damaged by sharp probes which can make holes and encourage the progression of lesions because plaque may now be difficult to remove (Figure 2.9). It is however, useful to draw a sharp probe gently across the lesion surface to feel whether it is matt (active) or shiny (arrested) but the probe should not be used as a bayonet!

The white spot lesion is more obvious on a dry tooth, but the lesion visible on the wet tooth is deeper into the tissues than the lesion only visible once the enamel is dry. This is to do with porosity and the relative refractive indices of air, water, and enamel. Enamel has a refractive index of 1.62. When carious, porous enamel is wet, the spaces are filled with water, which has a refractive index of 1.33. The difference in refractive index affects the light scattering, and the lesion looks white. If the tooth is now dried, the water is replaced with air, which has a refractive index of 1.0. The difference in refractive index between the air and the enamel is greater than between the water and the enamel. This explains why the lesion looks more obvious, or an earlier lesion can be detected.

2.3.5 The shape of the lesion and its clinical implication

On a smooth surface the lesion is classically triangular in shape. It follows the direction of the enamel prisms and can be thought of as multiple individual lesions each at a different stage of progression. The central traverse, where the lesion is deepest, is the oldest and most advanced part of the lesion where the biofilm is thickest. The shape of the lesion and the activity of the lesion entirely reflect the specific environmental conditions of the overlying biofilm (Figure 2.5).

Occlusally, purely because of the sloping fissure walls and the direction of the enamel prisms, the lesion assumes an undermining character. This explains why in the more advanced lesion, where there appears to be a small hole in the tooth, something apparently so small on the surface can be so large when entered with a burr (Figure 2.9) Once a cavity forms on this surface it is rather like a Marmite pot, narrower at the top than at the base (Figure 2.10). Now the toothbrush cannot reach into the hole to remove the plaque and the lesion is bound to progress.

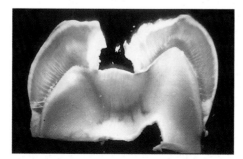

Figure 2.10. A hemisected occlusal lesion where there is a cavity in the tooth down to the dentine. At this stage the lesion spreads laterally along the enamel-dentine junction. Notice the shape of the cavity. It is wider at the base than at the top. This would prevent the patient cleaning plaque out of the hole.

2.4 DENTINE REACTIONS

The dentine has been reacting to the carious process in the biofilm long before a cavity forms. Dentine is a vital tissue, permeated by the tubules containing the cell processes of the odontoblasts, and it defends itself by the **tubular sclerosis** within the dentine and the formation of **tertiary dentine** (also called reactionary dentine or reparative dentine) at the pulp-dentine border (Figure 2.11).

Tubular sclerosis is the deposition of mineral within the dentinal tubules and it requires the presence of a vital odontoblast. It can be seen in the light microscope where a traverse through the centre of the enamel lesion crosses the enamel–dentine junction. The enamel demineralization has increased the enamel porosity and permeability and this dentine reaction corresponds to the most porous part of the enamel lesion, which in turn corresponds to the activity of the biofilm (Figure 2.12).

When contact between the enamel lesion and the enamel–dentine junction is established, the first sign of dentine demineralization can be seen along the junction as a brownish discolouration within the contact area of the enamel lesion and the junction. Demineralization of outer dentine is now surrounded by sclerotic reactions corresponding to the less advanced peripheral parts of the enamel lesion. Once again the dentinal changes merely represent a continuum of pulpodentinal reactions to the activity of the biofilm and transmission of the stimulus through the enamel in the direction of the enamel prisms. This means that regular disturbance or removal of the biofilm will arrest the progression of lesions, but the demineralized dentine remains as a scar in the tissue. It is very important to realize

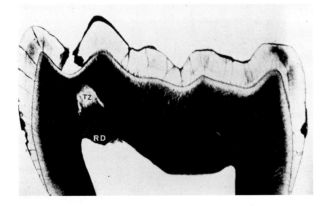

Figure 2.11. A ground section of a molar crown viewed in transmitted light. A fissure lesion is present. The enamel is cavitated. Tubular sclerosis is seen as a translucent zone in the dentine (TZ). Reactionary dentine (RD) is also present since the pulp horn is partially obliterated. (By courtesy of Professor N. W. Johnson.)

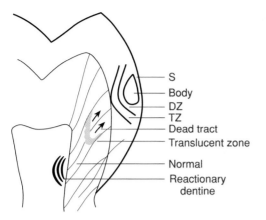

Figure 2.12. Diagram of histological changes in enamel and dentine before cavitation of the enamel. S, Surface zone; Body, body of lesion; DZ, dark zone; TZ, translucent zone. (By courtesy of Professor N. W. Johnson.)

that this dentine involvement *per se* is not an indicator for operative treatment. This dentine involvement is not actually an important moment clinically, but part of a continuum of changes all driven by the biofilm at the tooth surface.

2.5 CAVITATION—AN IMPORTANT MOMENT CLINICALLY

The important moment clinically may be the breakdown of the outer enamel, presumably created by mechanical injuries during mastication, micro-traumas during interdental wear, or careless probing. It is important because now it may be difficult to clean the biofilm out of the cavity (Figure 2.10). This protected area results in an ecological shift towards anaerobic and acid-producing bacteria. Once the biofilm is sitting on the dentine, demineralization can spread laterally along the enamel–dentine junction, undermining sound enamel (Figure 2.13).

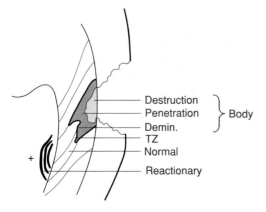

Figure 2.13. Diagram of histological changes after cavitation. Note that demineralization of enamel precedes bacterial penetration. TZ, translucent zone; DEMIN, demineralization. (By courtesy of Professor N. W. Johnson.)

2.6 DENTINE CHANGES IN THE CAVITATED LESION: DESTRUCTION AND DEFENCE

Following exposure of dentine to the mass of bacteria in the cavity, the most superficial part of the dentine is decomposed by the action of acids and proteolytic microorganisms. This is known as the **zone of destruction**. Beneath this, tubular invasion of bacteria is frequently seen which is called the **zone of penetration** because the tubules have become penetrated by microorganisms. Beyond this is an area of **demineralized dentine** which does not yet contain bacteria (Figure 2.13). When lesions progress rapidly, so-called **dead tracts** may form. Here the odontoblast processes have been destroyed without producing tubular sclerosis.

These tubules are invaded by bacteria and groups of tubules coalesce forming **liquefaction foci** (Figure 2.14). Destruction may also advance along the incremental lines of growth which are at right angles to the tubules to produce **transverse clefts** (Figure 2.15).

The defence reactions of tubular sclerosis and tertiary dentine formation continue as a response to these destructive processes. Both processes reduce the permeability of the dentine, although tertiary dentine is less well mineralized than primary or secondary dentine and contains irregular dentinal tubules. Even at this late stage removal of the mass of bacteria in the cavity, and/or placing a seal so the patient can clean, arrests the progression of

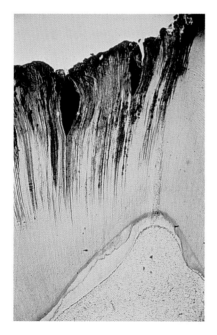

Figure 2.14. Decalcified section of carious dentine showing dentinal tubules penetrated by deeply staining bacteria. In places the tubules appear to have been pushed apart by aggregations of bacteria called liquefaction foci. (By courtesy of Professor N. W. Johnson.)

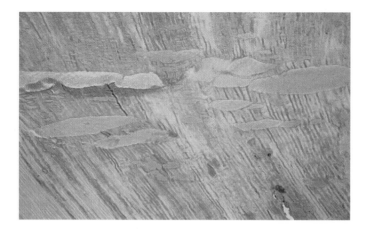

Figure 2.15. Decalcified section of carious dentine showing tubules penetrated by bacteria. The tissue appears to have split at right angles to the tubules along the incremental lines of growth. These splits are called transverse clefts. (By courtesy of Professor N. W. Johnson.)

lesions and encourages the two reparative processes. Even when dead tracts have formed and odontoblasts have been destroyed, new odontoblasts can form from fibroblasts in the pulp and lay down dentine. This is called **reparative dentine**. If the destructive processes continue, eventually the pulp becomes inflamed.

2.7 INFLAMMATION OF THE PULP

Inflammation is the fundamental response of all vascular connective tissues to injury. Inflammation of the pulp is called **pulpitis** and, as in any other tissue, it may be acute or chronic. The duration and intensity of the stimulus is partly responsible for the type of response. A low-grade, long-lasting stimulus may result in chronic inflammation whereas a sudden, severe stimulus is more likely to provoke an acute pulpitis.

In a slowly progressing carious lesion in dentine, the stimuli reaching the pulp are bacterial toxins and thermal and osmotic shocks from the external environment. The response to these low-grade, sustained stimuli is chronic inflammation which is well localized beneath the cavity. One rationale for restoring a cavity in a tooth is to remove or seal in the soft, infected dentine which is acting as an irritant, and fill the cavity with a restoration. The local inflammation then has the potential to repair. However, if the carious process continues, the organisms actually reach the pulp to create a 'carious exposure', and now localized acute inflammation is likely to be superimposed on the chromic inflammation.

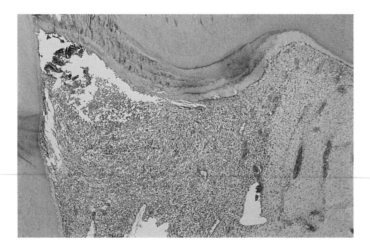

Figure 2.16. Chronic pulpitis as indicated by the tertiary (reactionary) dentine formation. A predominantly chronic (mononuclear) inflammatory infiltrate is gradually extending across and has largely replaced the normal coronal pulp tissue. (By courtesy of Professor R. Cawson.)

Inflammatory reactions have vascular and cellular components. The cellular component is most obvious in chronic inflammation (Figure 2.16) with lymphocytes, plasma cells, monocytes, and macrophages all present within the tissue. In time there may be increased collagen production leading to fibrosis. These chronic inflammatory reactions may not endanger the vitality of the tooth.

Unfortunately, the same cannot be said of acute inflammation, since in this process the vascular changes predominate, including dilation of blood vessels, producing an initial acceleration of blood flow and fluid exudate. This exudate may later result in retardation of blood flow and vascular stasis. There is active emigration of neutrophils (Figure 2.17) and all these factors contribute to an increase in tension of the tissue.

The outcome of this process is often localized necrosis, and in time this may involve the entire pulp. The sequel to pulpal necrosis is spread of inflammation into the periapical tissues (apical periodontitis). Once again, the inflammatory response may be acute or chronic.

2.7.1 Symptoms of pulpitis

Many studies have attempted to correlate the symptoms of which a patient complains with the level of inflammation in the pulp as determined by histological examination. These correlations are poor, and for this reason it is only possible to make some generalizations relating a patient's symptoms to the histological condition of the pulp.

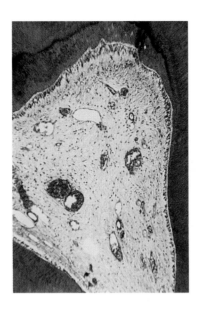

Figure 2.17. Early acute pulpitis showing the widely dilated pulp vessels and early emigration of leucocytes. There is patchy oedema of the dying odontoblast layer. (By courtesy of Professor R. Cawson.)

The first of these generalizations is that a chronically inflamed pulp is usually symptomless. In contrast, acute inflammation is almost always painful, the painful response being initiated by hot, cold, or sweet stimuli. Unfortunately the pain is often not well localized to the offending tooth, and the patient may not even be able to indicate which quadrant is involved.

What matters to the clinician is whether or not the pulp is likely to survive, because a pulp that will die should be removed and the pulp canal sealed with an inert filling material (root canal filling), or the tooth should be extracted. Since clinical symptoms relate so poorly to pulp pathology, there is an obvious problem here. A useful rule of thumb is to divide clinical pulpitis into reversible and irreversible pulpitis.

In **reversible pulpitis** the clinician hopes to be able to preserve a healthy vital pulp. The clinical diagnosis of reversible pulpitis is made when the pain evoked by a hot, cold, or sweet stimulus is of short duration, disappearing when the stimulus is removed. On the other hand, if pain persists for minutes or hours after removal of the stimulus, a clinical diagnosis of **irreversible pulpitis** may be made and the pulp removed and replaced by a root filling. Alternatively, the tooth may be extracted.

Whereas acutely inflamed pulps are painful, necrotic pulps are painless since there are no viable nerves to transmit pain. However, once the periapical tissues are involved, another set of symptoms may develop. Chronic periapical inflammation is usually painless, but acute periapical inflammation is often very uncomfortable, the pain being well localized. The inflammatory exudate is sometimes sufficient to raise the tooth slightly in its socket. Such a tooth is tender to bite on and tender to touch because it acts as a piston in its socket, transmitting forces directly to the inflamed periapical tissues. It is possible for acute periapical inflammation to become chronic and for chronic inflammation to become acute. The inflammation from acute periodontitis can spread to the adjacent soft tissues and produce a dramatic swelling. Eventually pus may discharge through a sinus: at this point pain is relieved, but inflammation may then become chronic.

2.8   THE MICROBIOLOGY OF DENTINE CARIES

The first wave of bacteria infecting the dentine is primarily acidogenic. Since demineralization precedes bacterial penetration, the acid presumably diffuses ahead of the organisms. The pH of carious dentine can be low, and members of the dentine bacterial community in active lesions tend to be acidogenic. When compared to the flora of supragingival plaque on intact enamel, infected dentine has higher proportions of Gram-positive bacteria. Thus lactobacilli predominate, with fewer mutans streptococci. The reasons for the ecological shift in the bacterial community could include the availability of the protein substrate and the low pH.

Within the zone of destruction there is a more mixed bacterial population, including organisms that can degrade the dentine collagen. This collagen degradation is preceded by demineralization of the mineral fractions of dentine.

These ecological shifts within the carious cavity may be of practical importance as well as academic interest. In the advanced dentine lesion what is driving the carious process? Is it the bacteria in the biofilm or the bacteria in the infected dentine, or both? The answer to this question is highly relevant to the operative management of carious dentine. Does carious dentine have to be removed in order to arrest the carious lesion?

Perhaps the lesion could be arrested by sealing off these organisms from the mouth. The reparative processes of tubular sclerosis and tertiary dentine would then also deprive them of nutrients from the pulp because the dentine is now less permeable to fluid exudate from the pulp. It is already known that sealing organisms in the tooth results in another ecological shift towards bacterial populations which are no longer cariogenic. These questions will be discussed again in Chapter 9.

2.9   ACTIVE AND ARRESTED LESIONS IN DENTINE

The rate of progress of caries in dentine is highly variable, and under suitable environmental conditions the carious process can be arrested and the lesion may even partly regress. Clinically, actively progressing lesions are soft and wet. Because of the speed of development of the lesion the defence reactions will not be well developed. Pain is easily evoked by hot, cold, and sweet stimuli. In contrast, arrested or slowly progressing lesions have a hard or leathery consistency. Histologically the defence reactions of tertiary dentine and tubular sclerosis are marked. The body of the lesion in dentine accumulates organic matter and mineral from oral fluids, the most striking remineralization taking place on and within a surface exposed to the oral environment.

It is very important to realize that even caries of dentine does not automatically progress. Before the enamel surface is cavitated these lesions can be arrested by preventive treatment. It is a dentist's responsibility to explain to patients how they may arrest the disease in their mouths.

2.10   ROOT CARIES

Up to now this chapter has considered caries of dentine beneath enamel caries. However, in many mouths root surfaces become exposed to the oral environment by gingival recession and these surfaces are now susceptible to root caries, and indeed are more vulnerable to mechanical and chemical destruction than enamel (Figure 1.5). Thus gingival recession is a prerequisite for exposure of a root surface, so it is hardly surprising that root caries is commonly seen in older people. It is associated with periodontal disease because this a major cause of gingival recession. However, this does not mean that all patients with exposed root surfaces will automatically get root caries, since cariogenic plaque is the essential prerequisite.

Clinically both active (soft) and arrested or slowly progressing lesions (hard or leathery) may be seen. Active lesions are usually close to the gingival margin in the area of plaque stagnation (Figure 1.5). Note it is the consistency of the lesion, rather than its colour, which is the guide to its activity.

Early root surface lesions have been shown on microradiographs (a radiograph of a ground section) to be radiolucent zones (i.e. zones of demineralization) below a well-mineralized surface layer which appears hypermineralized when compared with the neighbouring cementum. This hypermineralized surface zone covering early lesions is a consistent finding on exposed root surfaces but it is not present on non-exposed surfaces. This implies that mineral is likely to have precipitated from the saliva. Deep to the lesion there is frequently a hypermineralized area of tubular sclerosis and tertiary dentine is seen at the pulpal surface of the dentine corresponding to the involved tubules.

Destruction of apatite crystals thus appears to take place below the surface before bacteria penetrate into the root cementum and dentine. In this respect enamel caries and root caries are similar. However, bacteria seem to penetrate into the tissue at an earlier stage in root caries than in coronal caries. Root lesions are very vulnerable to mechanical damage, and probing with a sharp instrument should be almost totally avoided. It is also preferable to establish good plaque control but avoid root scaling until lesions have had the chance to arrest.

The recent dramatic decline in caries prevalence in children in many countries has resulted in an increased number of teeth being present in older individuals and for this reason root caries is of particular importance. The optimum management for root caries is again preventive treatment. Early diagnosis is important because active lesions may become arrested following improved plaque control with a fluoride toothpaste and care with diet. Root caries is particularly difficult to treat by operative means.

2.11 SECONDARY OR RECURRENT CARIES

Secondary or recurrent caries is **primary caries next to a filling** caused by the biofilm at the tooth surface or the surface of any cavity.

The histological picture will show primary caries next to the filling margin and there may be lines of demineralization, called wall lesions, running along the cavity wall. These are a consequence of leakage between the filling and the tooth, but clinical studies show this leakage does not lead to active caries beneath a filling.

2.12 RESIDUAL CARIES

Residual caries is demineralized and infected tissue left by a dentist during cavity preparation. There is no evidence that these entombed bacteria continue the carious process. When a filling is removed, residual caries is darkly

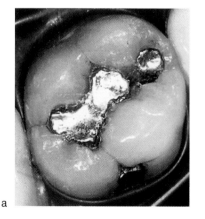 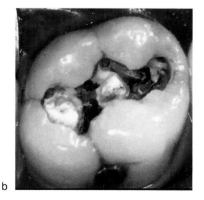

a   b

Figure 2.18. (a) This amalgam restoration has ditched margins and the enamel around the filling is stained. (b) The amalgam has now been dissected out of the cavity. The dentine beneath is stained brown and in places has a dry and crumbly texture. This is residual caries that the dentist left when the tooth was originally restored.

staining and either hard or dry and crumbly in texture (Figure 2.18). If cultured, few microorganisms are found.

When the filling was originally placed the dentine would have been soft, wet, and heavily infected. It is likely the organisms have died because their source of nutrient from the mouth has been cut off by the restoration, and from the pulp, by tubular sclerosis and tertiary dentine.

2.13 WHY IS DENTINE CARIES BROWN?

I do not know the answer to this! The possibilities seem to be:
- The colour is exogenous stain absorbed from the mouth (e.g. from tea, coffee, red wine).
- The colour comes from pigment-producing bacteria.
- The colour is the product of a chemical reaction called the Maillard reaction. A brown colour is produced when protein breaks down in the presence of sugar (think of cutting up an apple and leaving it).

Further reading

Fejerskov, O. and Kidd, E. A. M. (eds) (2003) *Dental Caries*. Ch. 5: Clinical and histological manifestations of dental caries. Blackwell Munksgaard, Oxford.

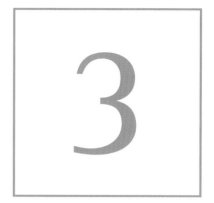

Caries diagnosis

3.1 INTRODUCTION

Diagnosis is identifying a disease from its signs and symptoms. The diagnosis of caries presents a number of traps for the unwary. First, there is the distinction made in Chapter 1 between the **carious process**, which occurs in the biofilm, and the reflection or symptom of this, the **carious lesion** on the tooth surface. The dentist sees the lesion which is the result of the metabolic activity in the biofilm but, paradoxically perhaps, has to remove plaque in order to see the lesion clearly. The trap would be to concentrate on the lesion without considering what makes the biofilm in this lesion, in this patient, conducive to progressive demineralization.

Another pitfall would be to **detect** demineralization without considering whether this is **active** and ongoing or already **arrested**. This information is important in terms of management. **Diagnosis** adds the aspect of activity to simple detection of lesions. However, it must also be remembered that caries diagnoses are always made in **conditions of uncertainty**. All diagnostic methods have inherent errors and it is just not possible to separate disease from no disease and active from arrested lesions. For one thing, the carious process is a continuum and it is not easy to judge where a particular lesion or patient lies on that continuous scale.[1]

It must also be appreciated that diagnostic tests needs to be both **valid** and **reliable**. Validity means that the test measures what it is intended to measure, e.g. a white spot lesion with a matt surface indicates an active lesion which has not yet cavitated. Reliability or reproducibility means the test can be repeated with the same result, e.g. the dentist would consistently recognize the same white spot lesion with a matt surface as an active lesion. The person should be consistent with himself or herself (intra-examiner reproducibility) and consistent with others (inter-examiner reproducibility).[2]

This seems to ask a lot, but it should be remembered that the dentist sees patients on recall. It is thus possible to make a diagnosis, take appropriate action and the **reassess** at a subsequent visit.[1]

3.2 WHY IS DIAGNOSIS IMPORTANT?

Diagnosis is important for three reasons:[2]
- It forms the basis for a treatment decision. Active lesions require some form of active management whereas arrested lesions do not.
- Informing the patient. The patient is central to the management of the carious process. It is the patient who will control the process, not the professional. The dentist's role is to inform the patient whether any action is required.
- Advising health service planners. Epidemiological surveys inform the politicians who commission them of the state of health and disease of the population. These surveys should assist them to direct money appropriately.

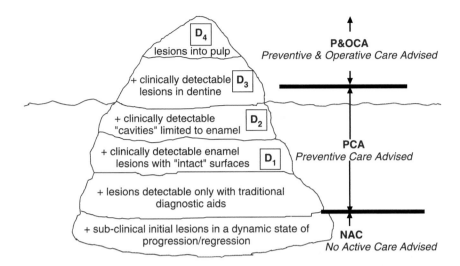

Figure 3.1. The 'iceberg of dental caries'. Diagnostic thresholds used in epidemiology and practice. In epidemiological surveys the iceberg 'floats' at the D3 threshold (cavity in dentine). Most lesions arrestable by preventive care are hidden below the water. If patients who only present with D1 and D2 lesions are described as 'caries-free' by epidemiologists, the politicians who commission the surveys will not appreciate the amount of preventive care the population requires. (Reproduced by kind permission of Professor Nigel Pitts.)

3.3 LEVELS OF DISEASE AND DIAGNOSIS[3]

Carious lesions may be diagnosed at any level of the carious process. For convenience the levels are graded D (for decay) followed by a number. The higher the number, the more advanced the lesion. Thus:
- D1 are clinically detectable enamel lesions with intact surfaces
- D2 are clinically detectable cavities limited to enamel
- D3 are clinically detectable lesions in dentine
- D4 are lesions into the pulp.

The more diagnostic aids that are applied and the more refined the methods, the more lesions will usually be identified. The hierarchy of these decisions and their relationship to the management required, have been elegantly represented as an iceberg (Figure 3.1). The diagnostic threshold can be thought of as the level at which the iceberg floats in the water.[3]

There is no universal diagnostic threshold that can be recommended for all purposes. For the dentist in the surgery the D1 threshold (enamel lesion, no cavity) is appropriate. This stage allows non-operative, preventive treatments which, if successful, should arrest the lesion. In epidemiological surveys (see page 13) diagnosis is at the D3 level, which inevitably underestimates the caries status by only recording lesions which are likely to require operative care. With contemporary knowledge of the carious process one must question whether it is appropriate for the survey epidemiologist to assess only the need for operative treatment.[3] This chapter will describe how the lesion can be diagnosed before, as well as after, the surface has cavitated.

3.4 PREREQUISITES FOR DETECTION AND DIAGNOSIS[2]

The diagnosis of caries requires **good lighting** and **dry, clean teeth**. If deposits of calculus or plaque are present, the mouth should be cleaned before attempting accurate diagnosis. Remember to brush plaque out of the fissures because it is easy to miss a white spot lesion at the entrance to a fissure unless the surface is clean (Figure 3.2). Do not remove plaque automatically, without thinking. After all, the process occurs within the plaque. Its presence or absence will be relevant to your decision about the activity of the lesion.

When the teeth have been cleaned, each quadrant of the mouth is isolated with cotton wool rolls to prevent saliva wetting the teeth once they have been dried. Thorough drying should be carried out with a gentle blast of air from the three-in-one syringe. White spot lesions are more obvious when teeth are dry (see page 29) and saliva can even obscure small cavities.

Sharp eyes can be used to look for the earliest signs of demineralization. Sharp probes should never be used to detect the 'tacky' feel of early cavitation, because a probe can damage a white spot lesion (see Figure 2.9) creating a hole which will subsequently trap plaque.

Good **bitewing radiographs** are also essential in diagnosis. In this technique the central beam of X-rays is positioned to pass at right angles to the long axis of the tooth, and tangentially through the contact area. The film is positioned in a film holder on the lingual side of the posterior teeth. The patient then closes the teeth together on the film holder. A beam-aiming

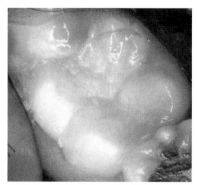 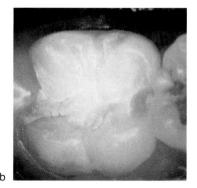

a   b

Figure 3.2. (a) This fissure looks both clean and caries free. It is not.
(b) The plaque has been brushed away and the surface has been dried. The lesion is now visible as white areas at the entrance to the fissure. (Reproduced by kind permission of *Dental Update*.)

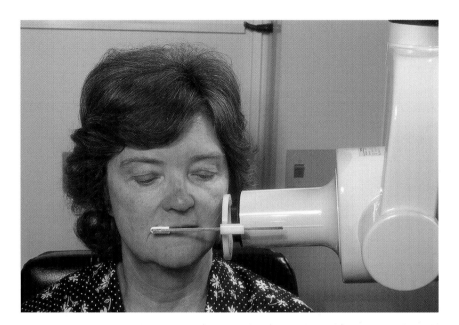

Figure 3.3. A bitewing radiograph is being taken. The film is held lingually by a film holder and the patient closes together on a part of this holder. A beam-aiming device helps the operator position the tube so that the beam is directed at right angles to the film.

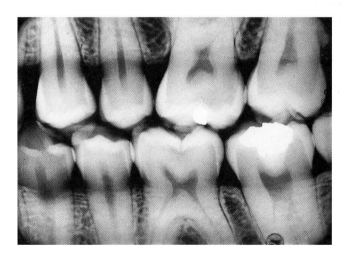

Figure 3.4. A bitewing radiograph showing occlusal caries in the lower first molar. Clinically there was no obvious cavity although the enamel was discoloured.

device on the holder guides the position of the tube (Figure 3.3). This directs the beam at right angles to the film and the contact areas of the teeth. The type of radiograph resulting can be seen in Figure 3.4.

3.5 DETECTION AND DIAGNOSIS ON INDIVIDUAL SURFACES[2]

3.5.1 Free smooth surfaces

Caries on free smooth **enamel** surfaces can be diagnosed with sharp eyes at the stage of the white or brown spot lesion (see Figures 1.4 and 2.7) before cavitation has occurred provided the teeth are clean, dry, and well lit. Drying is very important because, as explained on page 29, it gives the clinician an idea of the porosity and depth of the lesion. Active lesions tend to be plaque covered, close to the gingival margin and may have a matt appearance indicative of surface loss of tissue (see Figure 1.4 on page 6). These lesions may feel rough if the tip of a sharp probe is gently drawn across them (be gentle—the probe is an explorer, not a bayonet!). Arrested lesions, on the other hand, may have been abandoned by the gingival margin and may have a plaque free, shiny, lustrous surface (see Figure 2.2 on page 23). Sometimes these lesions are brown because the porosities have absorbed exogenous stain from the mouth.

Root surface caries, in its early stages, appears as one or more small, well defined, discoloured areas located in an area of plaque stagnation close to the gingival margin (Figure 3.5). Lesions may vary in colour from yellowish or light brown, through mid-brown to almost black. Active lesions are plaque covered, soft or leathery in consistency and may be cavitated. Arrested lesions are hard and are often located in a plaque free area coronal to the gingival margin (Figure 3.6). Arrested lesions may be cavitated.

Although lesion consistency is important in diagnosing activity, great care should be taken when using a sharp instrument on these surfaces. A

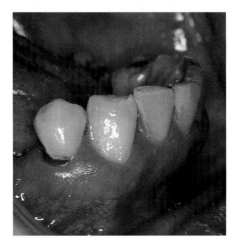

Figure 3.5. Root surface caries in an area of plaque stagnation close to the gingival margin.

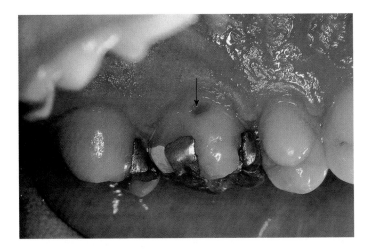

Figure 3.6. Arrested root caries in a plaque-free area, coronal to the gingival margin.

sharp probe could cause a small hole in which plaque will subsequently collect, possibly protected from the toothbrush bristle. It may be safer to test the consistency of the lesion by gentle use of a periodontal probe or the back of an excavator. It should be noted that colour is not a good indicator of lesion activity. It seems likely that the colour of the lesion is due to exogenous staining from such items as tea, coffee, red wine, or chlorhexidine mouthwashes. This colour may reflect the use of these liquids rather than lesion activity.

Root surface lesions tend to spread laterally and coalesce with minor neighbouring lesions and may thus eventually encircle the tooth. Commonly, the lesions extend only 0.25–1 mm in depth. They do not always spread apically as the gingival margin recedes, but new lesions may develop later at the level of the new gingival margin. This may occur irrespective of an arrested lesion being located more coronally at the cement-enamel junction of the tooth.

3.5.2 Pits and fissures (Figure 3.7)

Clinical-visual and radiographic examination

In order to carry out an accurate visual examination it is very important the surface is plaque free. Ideally the plaque should be disclosed and brushed away. Visual examination and examination of bitewing radiographs are both important. The active, uncavitated lesion is white, often with a matt surface. The corresponding inactive lesion may be brown. The enamel lesions are not visible on a bitewing radiograph. The enamel lesion that is only visible on a dry tooth surface is in the outer enamel. The lesion visible on a wet surface

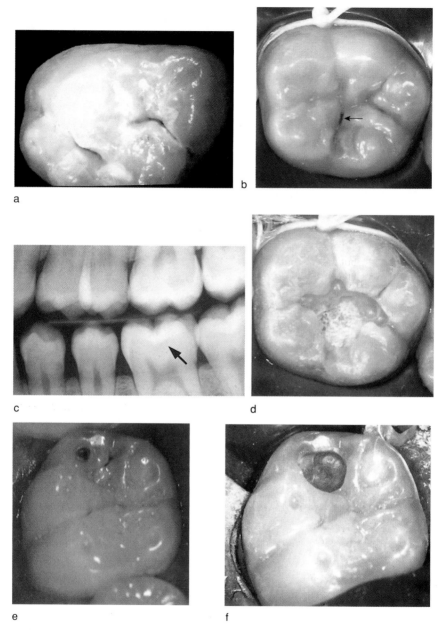

Figure 3.7. (a) White and brown spot lesions on the occlusal surface of a molar. There was no lesion in dentine on a bitewing radiograph. (b) A microcavity, looking like a slightly enlarged, brown fissure on a first lower molar (arrow). (c) A bitewing radiograph of the tooth seen in 3.7b shows occlusal caries in dentine (arrow). (d) The soft demineralized dentine has now been removed from the tooth seen in 3.7b–c. (e) An occlusal lesion in this molar is seen as a greyish discolouration of the enamel. This lesion was visible in dentine on a bitewing radiograph. (f) The lesion seen in 3.7e has now been accessed with an air rotor. Soft, demineralized dentine is present.

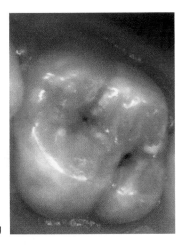
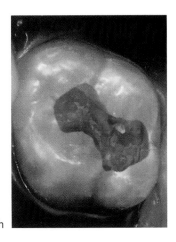

g

h

Figure 3.7. (g) Cavitated occlusal lesion is a first molar. The more mesial is a microcavity but the cavity on the distal aspect exposes dentine. The lesion was visible on a bitewing radiograph. (h) The lesion seen in 3.7g has now been accessed with an air rotor. This is a large lesion with much soft, demineralized dentine.

is all the way through enamel and may be into dentine. Cavitated lesions may present as microcavities with or without a greyish discoloration of the enamel. The microcavity is easily missed on visual examination. Careful examination of bitewing radiographs is important and serves as a useful safety net to avoid missing microcavities. A lesion that has been missed on visual examination but found on radiograph (Figure 3.4) has been called **hidden caries**. More advanced lesions may present as cavities exposing dentine. Cavitated lesions are usually visible in dentine on a bitewing radiograph. Cavitated occlusal lesions, whether microcavities or cavities down to dentine, are usually active because the patient cannot clean plaque out of the cavity (Figure 2.10, page 29).

Laser fluorescence method[4]

In recent years a laser fluorescence machine has become commercially available (DIAGNOdent, KaVo, Biberach, Germany) to aid the detection of occlusal caries. The machine emits light with a wavelength of 655 nm and this is transported through a fibre bundle to the tip of a handpiece (Figure 3.8). The tip is placed against the tooth surface and rotated. The laser light will penetrate the tooth. Different fibres in the tip receive the reflected light and fluorescence from the lesion, thought to be produced from bacterial porphyrins. The received light is measured and its intensity is an indication of the size and depth of the carious lesion. The machine is not detecting mineral loss *per se*. The reproducibility of the machine has been shown to be very

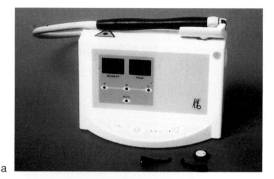

a

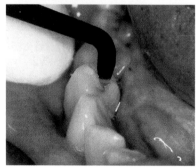

b

Figure 3.8. (a) The DIAGNOdent (KaVo, Biberach, Germany). (b) The machine in use with the tip on the occlusal surface of a premolar. The surface should be clean and dry.

good but it can be confused by staining and calculus, giving high readings when active caries is not present. Whether this machine will become a helpful tool in the diagnosis of occlusal caries when used by general practitioners has yet to be established. In the meantime, its readings should be interpreted with caution and combined with a conventional clinical-visual and radiographic examination.

3.5.3 Approximal surfaces[2]

Clinical-visual examination

It is difficult to see the white spot lesion on an approximal surface because the lesion forms just cervical to the contact area and vision is obscured by the adjacent tooth. The lesion is usually only discovered at a relatively late stage when it has already progressed into dentine and is seen as a pinkish-grey area shining up through the marginal ridge (Figure 1.3, page 5). It must be emphasized again that the teeth should be isolated, clean, and dry to see this.

In contrast, an approximal lesion on the root surface may be diagnosed visually but gingival health is mandatory for such a diagnosis to be reliable. Thus, if the gingivae are red, swollen, and tending to bleed, caries diagnosis in these areas should be deferred until improved oral hygiene has been instituted and the inflammation is resolved.

Tactile examination (careful!)

A sharp, curved probe (Briault) can be used gently to try to determine whether an approximal lesion is cavitated, but if this instrument or a scaler is used in a heavy-handed manner, it can actually cause cavitation.

Bitewing radiography

The bitewing radiograph is of paramount importance in the diagnosis of the approximal carious lesion (Figure 3.9), although it should be remembered that the technique is relatively insensitive as it is not able to detect early sub-surface demineralization. As shown diagrammatically in Figure 3.10, the approximal enamel lesion appears as a dark triangular area in the enamel of the bitewing radiograph. The lesion may be in the outer enamel or be seen throughout the depth of the enamel. Larger lesions can be seen as a radiolucency in the enamel and outer half of the dentine or a radiolucency in the enamel reaching to the inner half of the dentine. The pulp is often exposed by the carious process in this latter instance.

While the bitewing radiograph can detect demineralization, it cannot diagnose lesion activity. A series of radiographs taken over time are required to confirm the arrest or progression of lesions. It is essential that these views are geometrically comparable and the only reliable way to achieve this is to use film holders and beam-aiming devices (Figure 3.3).

Cavitated lesions are likely to be active because of the difficulty of removing plaque from the hole when an adjacent tooth is present. The presence or absence of a cavity cannot be judged from a radiograph but, referring

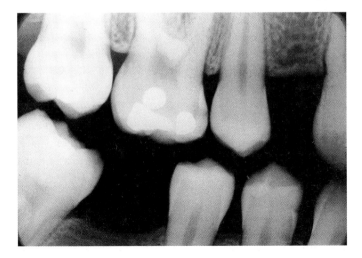

Figure 3.9. A bitewing radiograph showing caries in enamel and dentine on the mesial aspect of the upper first molar. A lesion is also visible on the mesial aspect of the lower first premolar.

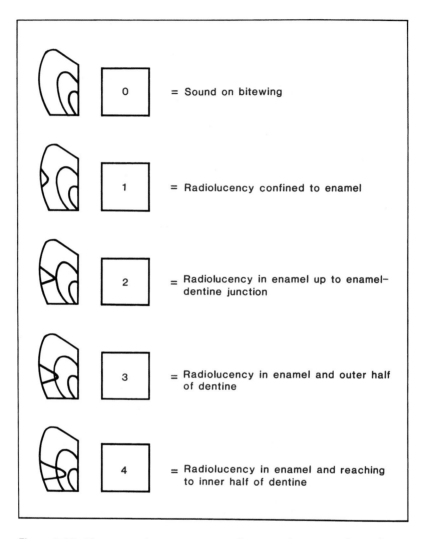

Figure 3.10. Diagrammatic representations of caries on bitewing radiographs.

to Figure 3.10, appearances graded 0–2 are unlikely to be cavitated, while grade 4 will almost certainly be cavitated. The problem comes with grade 3 which may or may not be cavitated. The dentist may wish to separate the teeth to determine whether a cavity is present and this technique is described on page 55.

Caries on the approximal root surface is also visible on a bitewing radiograph (Figure 3.11) although this appearance is sometimes confused with the cervical radiolucency. The latter is a perfectly normal appearance caused by the absence of the dense enamel cap at the enamel–cement junction and the absence of the interdental alveolar bone. Fortunately, root caries is

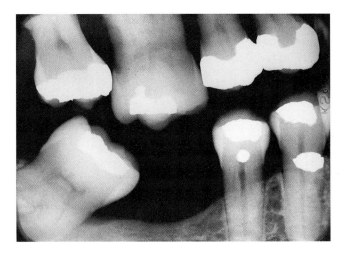

Figure 3.11. A bitewing radiograph showing root caries on the distal aspect of the first upper molar. This tooth has over-erupted following loss of the lower first molar.

visible clinically and a careful clinical re-examination will usually sort out any confusion.

It will be obvious that if it is to be of value, bitewing radiography must be carried out carefully. Overlapping contact points obscure what the clinician is trying to see and unfortunately, slight difference in angulation of the film or X-ray beam will affect what is seen on the resultant radiograph. Thus radiographs should be as reproducible as possible, using film holders with beam-aiming devices (Figure 3.3) and standardizing exposure time and dose. This is particularly important when the dentist is going to monitor lesions on radiographs over time to look for progression or arrest of lesions. In addition, films should be read dry, mounted, and under standardized lighting conditions.

Transmitted light

Transmitted light can also be of considerable assistance in the diagnosis of approximal caries. This technique consists of shining light through the contact point. A carious lesion has a lowered index of light transmission and therefore appears as a dark shadow that follows the outline of the decay through the dentine. The technique has been used for many years in the diagnosis of approximal lesions in anterior teeth. Light is reflected through the teeth using the dental mirror and carious lesions are readily seen in the mirror (Figure 3.12).

In posterior teeth a stronger light source is required and fibreoptic lights, with the beam reduced to 0.5 mm in diameter, have been used (Figure 3.13). It is important that the diameter of the light source is small so that glare

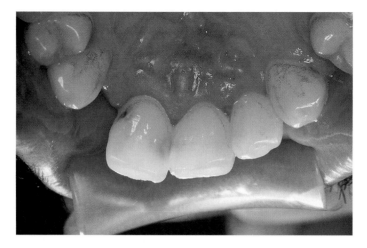

Figure 3.12. A mirror view of the palatal aspect of the upper anterior teeth. Lesions are visible mesially and distally on the upper right central incisor.

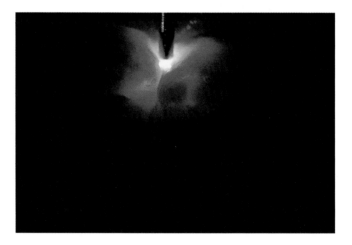

Figure 3.13. Use of a fibreoptic light in the diagnosis of approximal caries. (By courtesy of Professor C. Pine.)

and loss of surface detail are eliminated. The technique is called **fibreoptic transillumination** (FOTI). It has particular advantages in patients with posterior crowding where bitewing radiographs will produce overlapping images and in pregnant women where unnecessary radiation should be avoided.

Tooth separation

One further technique to assist with the diagnosis of approximal caries is the use of tooth separation. This technique has been borrowed from the ortho-

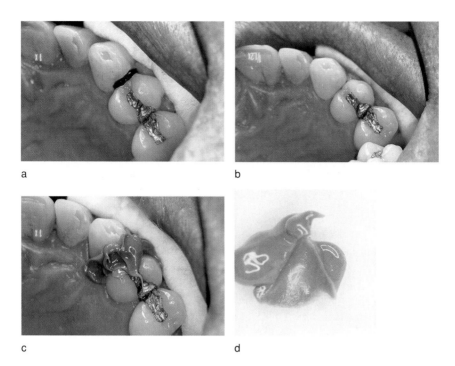

Figure 3.14. (a) Orthodontic separator is placed between the canine and first premolar. The dentist is unsure whether a restoration is required on the distal surface of the canine. On radiograph this surface shows a lesion through the enamel and clearly in dentine. (b) Separation achieved 48 hours later. Note it is not possible to see the distal surface of the canine clearly. (c) Taking an elastomer impression of the contact area. (d) Elastomer impression of the contact area showing no cavitation on the distal aspect of the canine; a restoration is not needed.

dontists who have used it for years to separate teeth before placing bands around them. A small round elastic is forced between the contact points using a special pair of applicating forceps (Figure 3.14a). After a few days the teeth are separated (Figure 3.14b). The dentist can now feel, very gently, with a probe to detect whether a cavity is present. Alternatively, a little elastomer impression material can be injected between the teeth(Figure 3.14c). After a few minutes the set material can be removed with a probe and the impression examined to see whether there is a cavity (Figure 3.14d).

3.5.4 Secondary or recurrent caries[2]

Secondary or recurrent caries is **primary caries at the margin of a restoration**. The clinical diagnostic criteria are thus identical to those for primary caries as described above.

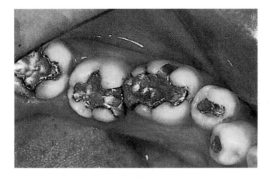

Figure 3.15. Ditched amalgam restorations.

Clinical-visual examination

A particular problem, with amalgam restorations is marginal breakdown or fracture, often called **ditching** (Figure 3.15). This has long been regarded with suspicion by clinicians, and restorations replaced as a preventive measure to avoid plaque stagnation in this area. There are a number of reasons why this approach is incorrect:

- Ditching occurs occlusally in an area that is easy to clean. Recurrent caries usually occurs approximally and cervically in areas of plaque stagnation.
- Clinical study has shown ditching does not reliably predict infected dentine beneath the ditched area unless the ditch is an obvious cavity that would admit the tip of a periodontal probe (over 0.4 mm).
- When dentists remove ditched fillings, they overcut cavities by as much as 0.6 mm. The dentist may also perpetuate the error of cavity preparation and restoration which caused the ditching problem. This is often too sharp an amalgam–margin angle, which makes the edge of the filling prone to fracture. The tooth is thus in danger of entering a repetitive restorative cycle until the dentist literally runs out of tooth tissue.

Discoloration around restorations with clinically intact margins also does not reliably predict new caries beneath the restoration (Figure 3.16). Sometimes discoloration around an amalgam can be caused by corrosion products from the amalgam or by light reflecting from the amalgam itself through the relatively translucent enamel. Discoloration around amalgam may also indicate demineralized, stained dentine, but this is residual caries left by the dentist who placed the filling. If these restorations are removed, the dentine is discoloured but either hard or crumbly and dry and not heavily infected. This does not indicate new disease. Staining around an amalgam restoration should not trigger its replacement unless a carious cavity, or a very wide ditch that traps plaque, is also present (Figure 3.17).

Colour changes around tooth-coloured filling materials may come in a number of forms. An active white spot lesion may be present and preventive treatment is indicated. A line of stain at the junction of the filling and the tooth may indicate leakage around the filling, but unless the patient requests its replacement because of poor appearance, operative treatment is not required (Figure 3.18).

Stain around a tooth-coloured filling can also present as grey or brown discoloured dentine shining up through intact enamel (Figure 3.19). This appearance probably represents residual caries left when the cavity was originally repaired. Clinical study indicates that this appearance does not reliably indicate

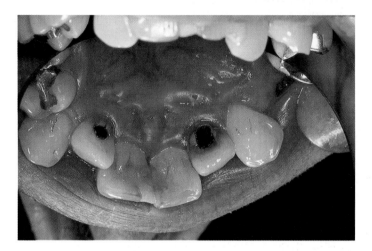

Figure 3.16. The enamel around the amalgam restorations on the palatal aspect of the upper lateral incisors is discoloured. Is this discoloration due to caries or corrosion of the amalgam? A decision was made to replace these restorations and removal of the amalgam revealed discoloured, hard, dentine. The replacement was unnecessary.

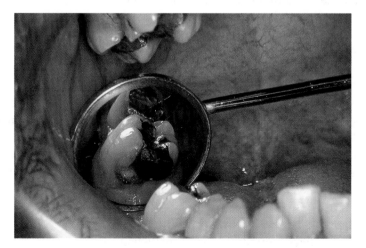

Figure 3.17. A cavitated carious lesion, full of plaque, is present at the cervical margin of the restoration in this molar.

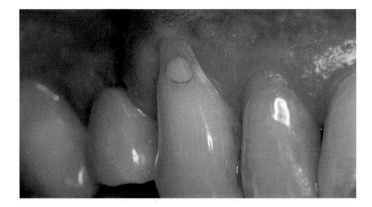

Figure 3.18. A line of stain at the junction of a tooth-coloured filling and the tooth.

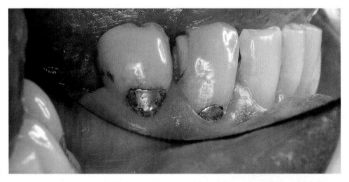

a

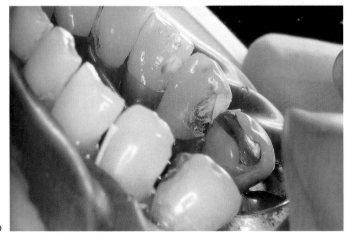

b

Figure 3.19. (a) Stained dentine around a tooth-coloured restoration.
(b) The appearance of the cavity once the restoration has been removed. Stained
and demineralized dentine can be seen. If this is either hard, or soft, dry, and
crumbly it is likely to be residual demineralization left when the restoration was
originally placed.

infected dentine (and presumably active demineralization) beneath the filling. If the margin of the filling is clinically intact it is unlikely that active caries is present beneath and the filling does not need to be replaced.

Bitewing radiographs

Bitewing radiographs are important in the diagnosis of recurrent caries because this usually occurs cervically in the area of plaque stagnation (Figure 3.20). It follows, therefore, that restorative materials should be radio-opaque.

Sometimes a radiolucency on radiograph indicates residual caries left when the restoration was placed. Figure 3.21 shows a bitewing radiograph of an amalgam restoration in a lower first molar with areas of radiodense dentine beneath the restoration. This appearance represents residual demineralized dentine left when the filling was originally placed. Tin and zinc ions from the amalgam have passed into the demineralized area to give the radiodense appearance. This restoration does not need to be replaced.

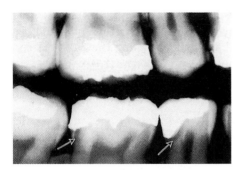

Figure 3.20. A bitewing radiograph showing root caries cervical to amalgam restorations. New restorations are indicated but preventive treatment is also very important.

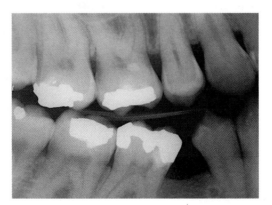

Figure 3.21. A large amalgam restoration is present in the lower first molar and areas of radiodense dentine are present beneath the approximal aspects of the filling. These areas probably represent residual demineralized dentine left when the cavity was originally prepared. Tin and zinc ions from the amalgam have passed into these areas to give the radiodense appearance.

3.6 DIAGNOSIS OF CARIES RISK[5]

The distribution of caries is highly uneven among contemporary populations. How convenient it would be if those at risk of developing carious lesions could be identified, both at the level of the individual in the surgery and the population. The dentist could then target expensive non-operative treatments appropriately and at a community level preventive efforts could also be targeted. This is called a 'high risk strategy'.

Although this concept seems both logical and laudable, it does not actually work. At the individual patient level, the best predictor of caries risk is current caries experience. Thus, the patient presenting with lesions is at risk of caries progression and developing new lesions.[5] This is obvious, but slightly frustrating because there is an element of 'shutting the stable door after the horse has bolted'!

To assess caries activity in an individual patient, note how many lesions are present (both cavitated and non-cavitated) and where they are located.[6] If a history of recent caries activity is available (number of lesions and fillings over the last 2–3 years) this is also valuable. A yearly increment of two or more lesions, detected clinically and/or radiographically, would indicate a high rate of lesion progression. The formation of lesions in areas such as lower incisors and buccal surfaces of molars, where salivary flow is relatively rapid, also indicates a high risk of caries progression.

3.7 EXPLAINING AN INDIVIDUAL'S CARIES EXPERIENCE[6]

Once a dentist has assessed a patient's caries activity status as high, an attempt should be made to identify the relevant risk factors because it may be possible to modify these and thus slow down disease progression. Some of these risk factors are listed in the box opposite.

3.7.1 Medical history

All patients should have their medical history taken, and this will include noting all medications. Some medications have sugar in their formulation, and if these are consumed frequently they can cause caries. In addition, some medications may decrease salivary flow. A low salivary flow rate predisposes to caries; the many reasons for this are discussed in more detail in Chapter 7. Each medication should be looked up in the British National Formulary because this lists the contents of the medication (including sugar) and whether the drug is known to cause a dry mouth.

Other diseases and treatments directly affect the salivary glands, such as Sjögren's syndrome and radiotherapy in the region of the salivary glands for head and neck malignancies.

FACTORS RELEVANT TO HIGH CARIES RISK

Medical history

Medications containing sugar

Medications known to cause a dry mouth

Radiotherapy for head and neck malignancy

Sjögren's syndrome

Disability

Dental history

History of multiple restorations

Frequent replacement of restorations

Sudden need for multiple restorations

Oral hygiene

Low frequency of tooth cleaning

Toothpaste that does not contain fluoride

Paste vigorously rinsed from the mouth?

Appliance worn e.g. orthodontic appliance; partial denture

Diet

Frequent sugary snacks or drinks

Fluoride

No fluoride supplementation e.g. no fluoride in toothpaste

Teeth rarely brushed

Saliva

Stimulated and unstimulated salivary flow is low

Social and demographic factors

Poverty

Low educational status

Unemployed

Religion and ethnicity may be relevant

Absence of fluoride in water

Those who are chronically sick may be unable to clean their mouths effectively. This is of particular importance in those who are in residential (nursing home) care because they can no longer look after themselves. Some patients with disabilities find oral hygiene difficult, and it is not always easy to obtain help with tooth cleaning.

3.7.2 Dental history

A history of multiple restorations and a need for frequent replacement of restorations is always relevant. These patients have proved themselves to be at high risk to caries, and dentist and patient need to work together to identify why this is. A sudden need for multiple restorations indicates something has changed. Perhaps it is salivary flow, perhaps diet, but again detective work is needed to try to identify the cause.

3.7.3 Oral hygiene

Since the carious process occurs in the plaque, questions about oral hygiene are very important. How often does the patient clean? How is the paste cleared from the mouth, by rinsing or spiting? Does the toothpaste contain fluoride? Is a mouthwash used? Does the patient use an appliance, such as an orthodontic appliance or a partial denture? These make cleaning more difficult and may increase caries risk (Figure 3.22). Plaque control and caries are considered further in Chapter 4.

3.7.4 Diet

Questions about diet are obligatory when a patient presents with active carious lesions or a history of multiple restorations that are frequently replaced. Dentist and patient are searching for an inappropriate dietary habit

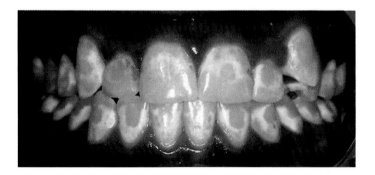

Figure 3.22. An orthodontist's nightmare! The brackets have been removed from the teeth and multiple white spot lesions have formed because oral hygiene was poor and many sugary snacks and drinks were consumed. The result is very unsightly.

which may partly explain the caries incidence. The detective process is explored further in Chapter 5.

3.7.5 Saliva

Saliva is a protective fluid as far as the mouth is concerned. A low secretion rate leads to reduced elimination of microorganisms and food remnants, impaired neutralization of acids, and a reduced ability to repair minor demineralizations. Increased caries activity is often seen in persons with a reduced rate of salivary secretion. However, although some patients are aware of a dry mouth (this is called **xerostomia**), others with reduced salivary flow (**hyposalivation**) do not realize they have a dry mouth. Dentists can sometimes detect a lack of saliva during the course of a clinical examination because the mouth mirror tends to stick to the mucosal surfaces or the saliva appears frothy.

Where a dry mouth is suspected, or in cases where a high caries incidence cannot be explained, stimulated and resting salivary flow rates should be measured. The normal secretion rates in adults are 1–2 ml/min for stimulated secretion and 0.3–0.5 ml/min for unstimulated secretion.

- **Stimulated salivary secretion rate.** The patient is asked to swallow any saliva present in the mouth and then to chew on a piece of paraffin wax. Saliva formed over the next 5 minutes is expectorated into a disposable cup. The volume of saliva secreted is measured by aspirating the saliva into a disposable graduated syringe (Figure 3.23). The secretion rate is

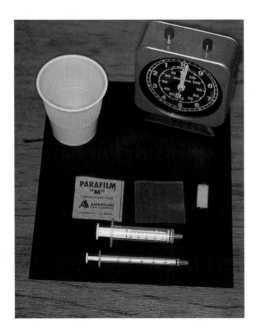

Figure 3.23. Paraffin film, paper cup, timer and disposable graduated syringes (1 and 5 ml) for measurement of salivary flow.

then expressed in millilitres per minute. When the secretion rate is very low, the saliva collected may also be frothy and difficult to measure. In such cases the addition of a measured amount of water will eliminate the froth and so facilitate measurement.

- **Unstimulated salivary secretion rate.** The patient sits quietly in the dental chair for 10 minutes, without chewing or swallowing but spitting into a disposable cup.
  - Normal unstimulated secretion rate in adults: 0.3–0.5 ml/min
  - Normal stimulated secretion rate in adults: 1–2 ml/min
  - Low stimulated secretion rate in adults: <0.7 ml/min
  - Severely dry mouth: <0.1 ml/min

Saliva is considered further in Chapter 7.

3.7.6 Social and demographic factors

These factors, although not directly involved in the carious process, can have an overriding influence in health and disease and on the changes in lifestyle a patient is able to make. It is not easy to assess these important issues, particularly when the patient is not in their home environment but on the dentist's territory, the dental surgery. Nevertheless the dentist will notice such things as cleanliness, age, dress, demeanour, disability, ethnicity, speech, educational status, and employment status. However, it is unwise to jump to conclusions, and relevant factors may only emerge after dentist and patient come to know each other better.

3.8 CATEGORIZING CARIES ACTIVITY STATUS[6]

Following history, clinical, and radiographic examination the dentist should categorize the patient as:

- **caries inactive**—no active lesions or history of recent restorations
- **caries active**—active lesions and or an annual increment of two or more new, progressing or filled lesions.

In the caries active patient it is sensible to try to list the factors that seem to be responsible. Some of these may be amenable to change, e.g. improving oral hygiene or diet. Others may be difficult to modify, e.g. an essential medication that also reduces salivary flow. Some factors may seem impossible to alter. Social factors such as poverty and education cannot be altered by the dentist. Behavioural factors may be very difficult to change, and these are discussed further in Chapter 8.

Further reading

1. Fejerskov, O. and Kidd, E. A. M. (eds) (2003) *Dental caries*. Ch.6: Caries diagnosis: 'a mental resting place on the way to intervention'? Blackwell Munksgaard, Oxford.
2. Fejerskov, O. and Kidd, E. A. M. (eds) (2003) *Dental caries*. Ch.7: Clinical and radiographic diagnosis. Blackwell Munksgaard, Oxford.

3. Fejerskov, O. and Kidd, E. A. M. (eds) (2003) *Dental caries.* Ch.9: Caries epidemiology with special emphasis on diagnostic standards. Blackwell Munksgaard, Oxford.
4. Fejerskov, O. and Kidd, E.A.M. (eds) (2003) *Dental caries.* Ch.8: Advanced methods of caries diagnosis and quantification. Blackwell Munksgaard, Oxford.
5. Fejerskov, O. and Kidd, E. A. M. (eds) (2003) *Dental caries.* Ch.22: Caries prediction. Blackwell Munksgaard, Oxford.
6. Fejerskov, O. and Kidd, E. A. M. (eds) (2003) *Dental caries.* Ch.20: Caries control for the individual patient. Blackwell Munksgaard, Oxford.

4

Prevention of caries by plaque control

4.1 INTRODUCTION

The carious process is the metabolic activity in the plaque (the biofilm). The result may be nothing to see or there may be a net loss of mineral resulting in a carious lesion that can be seen. **Plaque is the cause of caries, and a tooth which is completely free of plaque will not decay**.

However, it is not always possible to demonstrate a strong association between the presence of dental plaque and caries, and there are some obvious reasons for this. For one thing, people are not able to completely remove plaque themselves, even with supervision. In addition, although the bacterial biofilm is the cause of caries, there are other factors involved. This is why caries is described as a multifactorial disease. These factors may increase or decrease the rate of demineralization.

To give examples, increased sugar intake and decreased salivary flow speed up the carious process. On the other hand, fluoride tends to decrease the rate of mineral loss. Thus it is not only amount of plaque that matters but the combined effect of all the factors, and the combination of factors, which will vary from patient to patient.

Brushing twice daily with a fluoride toothpaste has been advocated by the profession for many years, and this behaviour is a routine part of many people's behaviour. This daily brushing with a fluoride toothpaste is believed to be the primary reason for the decline of caries observed in many populations since the 1970s. The behaviour should not be taken for granted. Patients should always be asked whether, and how often, they brush their teeth and what toothpaste they use. Most toothpastes contain fluoride, but not all, and it is important to check this. In UK a well-known brand of toothpaste for sensitive teeth is produced in a number of flavours, and at the time of writing, not all these products contain fluoride. Since cavities in teeth can be sensitive to hot and cold, it is not unusual for patients with caries to select a toothpaste for sensitive teeth. Thus the very person who most needs a fluoride toothpaste is sometimes not using it. Some herbal toothpastes are also formulated in a fluoride-free form.

4.2 EVIDENCE OF THE IMPORTANCE OF TOOTH CLEANING[1]

The designs of clinical studies to assess the caries preventive effect of toothbrushing vary greatly. Some will indicate whether the procedure **can** work, given full compliance by all concerned. Others are more pragmatic in design, trying to find out whether the procedure **does** work in a real-world community setting when some individuals comply and other do not. It is helpful to consider the evidence at different levels:
- an individual site
- individual patients
- the community.

4.2.1 The individual site

Strong evidence supporting the effect of oral hygiene on caries comes from experimental studies carried out *in vivo*. For instance, it was reported in 1970[2] that when dental students stopped brushing for 23 days white spots developed along gingival margins of teeth. Students who were in a group rinsing frequently with sucrose in the test period developed more lesions than those who did not rinse. But **all** lesions were reversible after 30 days of careful oral hygiene and daily fluoride mouth rinses (0.2% sodium fluoride).

In other studies plaque formation has been encouraged by placing bands onto teeth to encourage plaque stagnation beneath the band. White spot lesions developed over 4 weeks but when the bands were removed and tooth-brushing restarted, these lesions were no longer so obvious, apparently because of surface wear (see page 24).

A number of experiments on the role of plaque removal in caries control are carried out *in situ*. Here subjects carry slices of enamel or dentine, often on dentures. Sometimes the specimens contain carious lesions and the experiment monitors how they change with brushing. In other studies, lesions are created and then brushed or not brushed, to measure how they progress. The advantage of the *in situ* design is that the tooth slices can be examined histologically at no detriment to the patient.

Collectively these studies show it is possible to control the development and progression of carious lesions by meticulous oral hygiene with a fluoride toothpaste. This is very important information because it means that patients should be shown how to remove plaque over specific lesions. At a community level there may not be a strong association between plaque and caries. But to argue from this that plaque control is not important in caries management is biologically illogical and flies in the face of this individual site evidence.

4.2.2 The individual patient

Children whose dental cleanliness is consistently good may get less caries than those whose cleanliness is consistently bad. Several studies show participants brushing twice daily develop fewer lesions than those brushing less frequently. It is thus sensible to recommend that patients should brush twice daily with a fluoride toothpaste.

In most studies it is not possible to separate the effect of the brushing from the effect of the fluoride in the toothpaste. It would not now be considered ethical to have a group of volunteers brushing with a fluoride-free toothpaste. However, it is possible to look back to clinical studies comparing fluoride and non-fluoride toothpastes conducted in the 1960s and 1970s. These studies usually lasted 2–3 years, and in this rather short time period the fluoridated pastes showed a reduction in caries of about 24%.[3] Thus the effect of fluoride in the paste is very important.

The most simple and effective way to control the development and progression of caries at the individual level is to brush away plaque with a fluoride toothpaste.

4.2.3 The community

There is no clear-cut association between oral hygiene and caries in population studies but, as discussed in the introduction to this chapter, this is not surprising because caries is a multifactorial process. Another rather intriguing explanation may relate to the way plaque was measured in these studies. The indices used were developed for periodontal purposes and concentrate on gingival plaque which may be a poor predictor of caries because carious lesions form on occlusal and approximal surfaces and not only adjacent to gingival margins.

It is a mistake to look on toothbrushing as only a vehicle for fluoride application. The quality of plaque removal is also important at the individual site where a lesion is developing and to the individual patient. In addition, there is likely to be a synergistic effect between plaque and diet. It has been shown that the risk of caries increased with increasing levels of plaque at all levels of sugar consumption. Thus, when sugar consumption is high, plaque removal can help control the development and progression of caries.

4.24 Professional tooth cleaning

It is not always possible to get people to clean their teeth as well as they should. There are two possible difficulties:
• they are not sufficiently dextrous to do it
• they can, but they **will not**!

In an attempt to overcome these difficulties, two Swedish researchers, Axelsson and Lindhe, developed a professional tooth cleaning programme (the Karlstad programme).[4] In addition to the traditional components of a caries-preventive programme (repeated oral hygiene instruction, dietary advice, and topical fluorides) professional personnel cleaned the teeth at regular intervals. The idea was based on the study conducted in dental students that showed where dental plaque was allowed to accumulate on a clean tooth surface, white spot lesions developed in the enamel in 2–3 weeks. Thus plaque was removed professionally from all tooth surfaces every 2 weeks, together with a topical application of fluoride, to control caries. Children in the control group undertook supervised brushing at school, once every month, with a fluoride solution.

When this programme was carried out in children every 2 weeks during the school term, the results were dramatic, the number of lesions per year reducing from 3 per child to a single lesion in every 10 children. Later studies by the Karlstad group showed the caries-controlling effect could be retained in well-motivated children and adults, despite increasing intervals between appointments up to 3 months.

Researchers who have applied this method in other populations have not always obtained such impressive results but it does appear particularly effective on tooth surfaces that are difficult to clean, such as approximal surfaces and erupting occlusal surfaces. This is a highly expensive treatment programme, but it may be justified in the management of some highly caries active patients.

4.3   MECHANICAL REMOVAL OF PLAQUE

The quality of toothbrushing is very important to its caries preventive effect. The aim of this section is to help the professional advise the patient how best to remove plaque.

4.3.1 Seeing plaque: disclosing agents and mirrors

In order to learn how to remove plaque effectively, it is helpful for the patient to see where it is present. Since plaque is translucent and has a colour similar to teeth, it must be stained in order to be seen clearly (see Figure 1.1, page 2). Liquids, tablets, or capsules containing erythrosine or vegetable dyes, called **disclosing agents**, are used to stain plaque. Once a patient has been taught to identify plaque, the disclosing agent should be applied after toothbrushing so that areas where oral hygiene is inadequate can be seen easily. However, it will only be possible if the bathroom mirror used at home by the patient is well illuminated and a mouth mirror is also used. An inexpensive magnifying shaving mirror together with a disposable mouth mirror (Figure 4.1) are invaluable aids for effective oral hygiene. When adequate lighting is a problem, a mirror–light combination is a good solution.

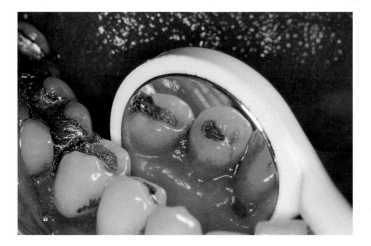

Figure 4.1. A disposable mouth mirror allows the patient to see plaque on lingual and interproximal areas.

4.3.2 Toothbrushes

Manual toothbrushes

Toothbrushes vary widely in shape and size of the head, the material, texture, and arrangement of filaments as well as in the size and shape of the handles. In general it is accepted that brushes should have:

- a handle appropriate to the age and dexterity of the user
- a head size appropriate to the user's mouth; a brush with a small head is generally recommended
- a compact arrangement of medium hard, rounded nylon filaments
- a bristle pattern which enhances plaque removal; brushes with bristles arranged at different heights and angles are available, and some studies have shown these are more effective than flat-trim brushes in removing plaque and reducing gingivitis.

What matters is that the brush chosen by the patient should be effective for them. Thus the professional should only institute change if they perceive a problem. It is important that brushes are replaced regularly, at least every 3 months, or sooner if the bristles become permanently bent. A brush that shows signs of wear cannot clean effectively.

Although there is considerable variation in manual dexterity, most healthy individuals can be taught to clean their teeth effectively, provided they are sufficiently motivated. However, for many patients, especially the physically handicapped where manual dexterity is limited, a powered toothbrush is very useful.

Powered toothbrushes

Most modern powered toothbrushes have a small, circular head which performs oscillating, rotating, or counter-rotational movements (Figure 4.2). Some models have timers which give useful feedback to the user on the time they have spent brushing.

A recent review of evidence[5] concluded that powered toothbrushes with an oscillating/rotating movement were more effective in removing plaque

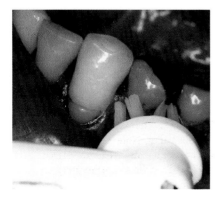

Figure 4.2. A powered toothbrush with a small, circular head which performs rotating movements.

and reducing gingivitis than manual brushes. It has also been reported that powered toothbrushes improve compliance.

4.3.3 Methods of toothbrushing

Various methods of toothbrushing have been advocated and classified according to the type of motion performed by the brush:
- the **scrub** method is performed by using a horizontal scrubbing motion and is usually recommended for children and for occlusal surfaces of teeth
- in the **Bass** method a vibratory motion is used.

In reality it does not matter exactly how a toothbrush is used, as long as plaque is removed effectively without trauma to the gingival tissues. Disclosing agents will show areas where plaque removal is ineffective. The patient should now be asked to clean these areas as they would normally. Where plaque still persists, the professional should teach effective oral hygiene. The recommended method will depend upon the dexterity of the individual patient as well as configuration of the teeth. The vibratory Bass technique is the most useful and will be described in detail.

The Bass method (Figure 4.3)

The brush is held so that the bristles are directed apically and then placed against the gingival margin at an angle of 45° to the long axis of the tooth. The brush is pressed so that the bristles are flexed and the tips forced between the teeth. It is then vibrated either in an anterior–posterior direction or by a rotary movement of the handle, keeping the tips of the bristles in position. This method of brushing is advocated in patients with open interdental spaces because it facilitates the penetration of the brush filaments. In order to clean the lingual surfaces of the upper and lower anterior teeth the brush may have to be turned into a vertical position, using the bristles at the 'toe' of the brush to obtain proper access to the gingival area of the teeth.

The Bass method is effective in removing plaque adjacent to and directly below the gingival margin. Since the bristles of the brush are directed

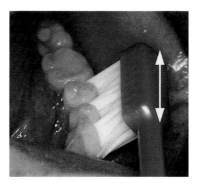

Figure 4.3. The Bass method of toothbrushing. Note the angulation of the bristles against the tooth surface and the direction of the vibratory motion.

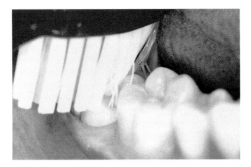

Figure 4.4. Cleaning a partly erupted tooth with a toothbrush. The parent should stand behind the child and bring the brush in at right angles to the arch. (By courtesy of *Dental Update*).

towards the gingival tissues and may be potentially damaging, a hard brush must not be used with this method.

Some patients will pick up a new cleaning technique easily, while others find it difficult. It is sometimes helpful to guide the patient's hand so that they can feel the motion required.

Occlusal surfaces

A horizontal scrubbing motion should be used on occlusal surfaces. When teeth are erupting they are below the level of the occlusal plane and must be cleaned individually by bringing the toothbrush in at right angles to the arch (Figure 4.4). With the erupting first molars the child (aged about 6 years) needs help to get these surfaces perfectly plaque-free. The helper should stand behind the child to 'finish off' their brushing. Molar teeth can take as long as 2 years to erupt, and this is a critical time as far as caries is concerned.

4.3.4 Interdental cleaning

Approximal surfaces and areas where teeth are malaligned cannot be reached with an ordinary toothbrush. Consequently, additional aids such as dental floss or tape, single-tufted brushes, or interdental brushes may be required for these areas. Choice will depend on the shape of the interdental area and the dexterity of the individual.

Dental floss or tape

In a young and healthy mouth, where the interdental papillae fill the interdental spaces, the use of dental floss or tape is the method of choice for interproximal cleaning. No differences have been found in cleansing potential between waxed and unwaxed floss, although unwaxed floss tends to fray more readily. Ribbon floss or tape is wider than ordinary floss and seems to be easier to use.

It is necessary to teach the patient the correct technique for applying floss, otherwise damage to the gingival tissues is likely. The correct technique illustrated in Figures 4.5 and 4.6. The fingers holding the floss should not be

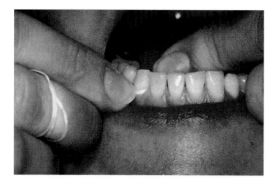

Figure 4.5. The use of dental tape for interproximal cleaning of the lower teeth. Two index fingers are used to control the floss.

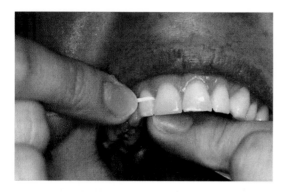

Figure 4.6. The use of dental tape for interproximal cleaning of the upper teeth. Note how the controlling fingers are close together and the tape is wrapped around the surface of the tooth being cleaned.

more than half an inch apart. The floss should be guided slowly through the contact point and then wrapped around the interproximal surface of each tooth in turn. A vertical, up and down motion along the surface is then used to remove plaque. The index fingers of both hands are usually used to control the floss (Figures 4.5, 4.6). For the upper teeth it may be easier to use the index finger of one hand and the thumb of the other hand. A clean section of floss should be used for each interproximal space. Patients who are sufficiently motivated can usually learn to floss adequately, although some patients take longer to grasp the technique. In such patients floss holders may be helpful (Figure 4.7).

'Super' floss (see also Figure 4.7) is specially designed to clean under bridgework. A section of the floss, about 12 cm long, is thickened with a foamlike material and when threaded under a bridge is very effective in removing plaque (Figure 4.8).

Interdental brushes
When there are wide interdental spaces present an interdental brush is ideal for the removal of interdental plaque (Figure 4.9). It is also a useful aid for

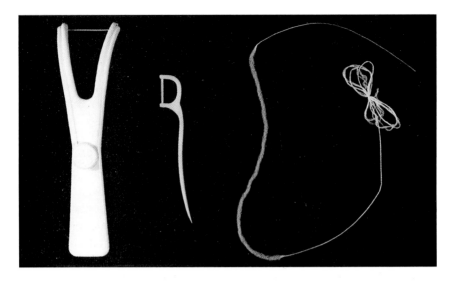

Figure 4.7. Floss holders and 'Super' floss.

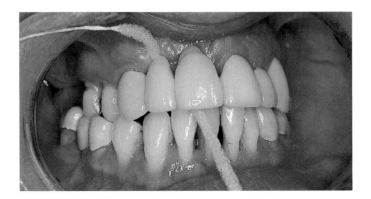

Figure 4.8. The use of 'Super' floss to remove plaque under a bridge.

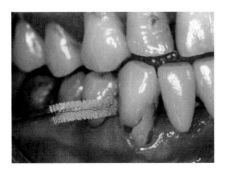

Figure 4.9. The use of an interdental brush.

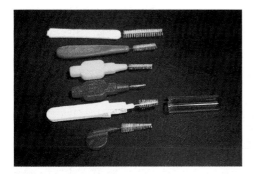

Figure 4.10. Interdental brushes in various sizes.

cleaning around bridges. This brush is shaped like a miniature bottle brush and is available in different sizes (see Figure 4.10). The smaller brushes are usually inserted into handles to make them easier to manipulate. It is important to select the correct size of brush to fit the particular interdental space to be cleaned. It is also important to 'see the patient in action' to be sure they are using it correctly.

Single-tufted brushes

It is often difficult to reach the distal surfaces of posterior teeth or areas where teeth are malaligned. A single-tufted brush (Figure 4.11) is a very useful additional aid for cleaning these areas.

4.3.5 Toothpastes

In the past toothpastes were used in conjunction with a toothbrush solely for cosmetic and social reasons. However, in the last 30 years fluorides, antibiotics, ammonium compounds, enzyme inhibitors, and bicarbonate have been added in attempts to inhibit dental caries. Of all these agents, only fluoride has stood up to clinical testing for safety and efficacy in caries prevention. It is also becoming increasingly common for manufacturers to add other therapeutic or preventive agents to reduce gingivitis and calculus formation. A few toothpastes also contain desensitizing agents. Although the line between the cosmetic and therapeutic actions is not easily drawn, most

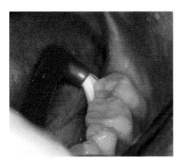

Figure 4.11. The use of a single-tufted brush for cleaning the lingual surface of a lower molar.

toothpastes currently on sale have similar objectives. They clean and polish the accessible surfaces of the teeth and provide a pleasant sensation and odour to the oral cavity. They also act as a vehicle for applying fluoride to tooth structure.

Composition of toothpastes

Most toothpastes are produced in paste form and have a similar basic formulation. A few powder dentifrices are available containing abrasives, detergents, flavouring, colouring agents, and sweeteners. Toothpastes contain all these agents as well as binding agents, humectants, preservatives and water. Most toothpastes in the UK and the USA contain fluoride, and many pastes also contain other therapeutic or preventive agents.

The constituents of toothpaste and their functions are as follows:

Cleaning and polishing agents (30–40%)

These abrasive agents are the major constituents of toothpastes and may consist of silica, calcium carbonate, dicalcium phosphate, sodium metaphosphate, hydrated alumina, zirconium silicate, or calcium pyrophosphate.

There is considerable variation in the inherent abrasivity of toothpastes, depending upon which abrasive system is used. However, the hardness of the toothbrush and the force used may also affect the actual abrasion experienced. All toothpastes sold in the UK must not exceed a specified level of abrasivity set by the British Standards Institute. In practice, most dentifrices will remove plaque and pellicle without removing significant amounts of enamel. However, if a hard brush is used with force, particularly on exposed root surfaces, abrasion can cause serious loss of dental tissue.

Detergents (1–2%)

The purpose of these agents is to facilitate the distribution of the paste in the mouth by lowering the surface tension and helping to loosen plaque and other debris from the tooth surface. They also contribute to the foaming action of toothpastes. The detergents commonly used are sodium lauryl sulphate and sodium N-lauryl sarcosinate.

Binding agents (1–5%)

Alginates, gums, or cellulose derivatives such as carboxymethyl cellulose and hydroxyethyl cellulose are used to prevent separation of the solid and liquid ingredients during storage.

Humectants (10–30%)

These agents are used to retain moisture and prevent hardening of the paste on exposure to air. Glycerol, sorbitol, and propylene glycol are commonly used.

Flavouring and sweetening agents (1–5%)

The taste of a toothpaste is one of its most important selling points. In order to mask the less pleasant taste of some of the other ingredients, flavouring agents such as aromatic oils (peppermint, spearmint, cinnamon, winter-green) and menthol are added. The glycerol and sorbitol, used as humec-tants, sweeten the paste. In addition, saccharin may also be used.

Preservatives (0.05–0.5%)

Alcohols, benzoates, formaldehyde, and dichlorinated phenols are added to the toothpaste in order to prevent bacterial growth on the organic binders and humectants.

Colouring agents

These are added to make the product look attractive.

Therapeutic and preventive agents

Many toothpastes now contain therapeutic and/or preventive agents for specific problems. In order to be effective it is important that these agents do not react with the other constituents of the paste.

• *Fluorides*

The caries-reducing effect of toothpaste containing fluoride is in the region of 24%.[3] In Europe, toothpastes containing a maximum concentration of 1500 ppm are on general sale as cosmetic products. Formulations with higher concentrations are available as prescription-only medicines. Fluoride concentration is an important determinant of anticaries efficancy.[6]

Low-fluoride toothpastes, containing less than 600 ppm of fluoride, are available for young children in the UK. However, these low-fluoride tooth-pastes provide less protection than those containing higher concentrations. The choice of fluoride concentration is considered further in Chapter 6, page 118.

• *Desensitizing agents*

Toothpastes formulated to alleviate sensitivity of exposed dentine contain one of the following agents: strontium chloride, strontium acetate, formal-dehyde, potassium nitrate and chloride, or sodium citrate.

• *Antiplaque agents*

Several toothpastes contain tricolsan, an antibacterial agent that is non-ionic (i.e. it has no charge). Unlike other proven cationic (positively charged) plaque-inhibiting agents such as chlorhexidine, triclosan does not react with the detergents in the dentifrice. Because it is non-ionic its retention in the mouth is poor, but this has been enhanced by combining it with a copolymer or boosting its antibacterial activity with zinc citrate. Such triclosan-containing toothpastes have been shown to reduce plaque formation and gingivitis to some extent. A clinical trial demonstrated that the triclosan/ copolymer/fluoride formulation gave similar caries protection when compared with fluoride control.

An oxygenating system using the enzymes amyloglucosidase, and glucose oxidase has been added to a toothpaste to stimulate salivary peroxidase. Theoretically, this, in turn, increases production of hypothiocyanite which has antibacterial properties. However, studies assessing the plaque-inhibiting effects of toothpastes containing the enzymes have produced conflicting results.

• *Anticalculus agents*
Several different agents have been added to reduce the formation of supragingival calculus. These include pyrophosphates, diphosphonates, zinc salts, and Gantrez acid (a copolymer of methyl ether and maleic anhydride). Calculus reductions reported for the various systems range between 10 and 50%.

• *Bicarbonate*
Bicarbonate has been added to toothpaste. The rationale for its inclusion is that it is alkaline and may, therefore, reduce the acidity of dental plaque. This would create a hostile environment for the growth of aciduric bacteria such as mutans streptococci and lactobacilli. There are no reported clinical trials of these formulations in relation to caries in humans at present.

• *Xylitol*
This sugar alcohol, which cannot be fermented by oral microorganisms, is added to some toothpaste in Scandinavia. It sweetens the paste and it may have an anticaries action by enhancing remineralization and reducing the levels of mutans streptococci.

• *Mucosal irritation due to dentifrices*
A small percentage of individuals are sensitive to some of the ingredients of dentifrices, particularly the aromatic oils. This can be expressed as desquamation or ulceration of the oral mucosal, gingivitis, angular cheilitis, and perioral dermatitis. Patients with dry mouths find strongly flavoured toothpastes particularly uncomfortable. The practical solution to this problem is for the patient to change to another dentifrice with a different flavour. Ideally, these patients should use a flavourless paste but unfortunately such a toothpaste is not yet commercially available.

4.3.6 Professional plaque control

In caries-active patients who for some reason do not master plaque control themselves and/or in patients with decreased salivary secretion (less than 0.3 ml/min; see page 63) additional plaque control in the form of professional tooth cleaning can give the patient some extra support.

The clinical procedure is as follows:

- Disclose plaque.
- Remove plaque with a low abrasive, fluoride-containing polishing paste. A handpiece (rotating up to 5000 rpm) is used with a pointed bristle brush for the fissures and a rubber cup for free, smooth surfaces. For proximal surfaces the paste is applied with a toothpick or interdental brush. Floss all contacts to ensure though plaque removal.
- Disclose again and check that all plaque has been removed.
- Apply Duraphat varnish to sites with active lesions. Duraphat contains sodium fluoride in an alcoholic solution of natural varnishes. It is ideally applied on clean, dry teeth with a brush or sponge applicator but will cling on to teeth even if moisture is present. The varnish has a high fluoride concentration (22 mg/ml) and is contra-indicated in children under 6 years who may swallow some of the product.
- Review the patient every 2–3 weeks initially. Always start these visits with disclosing and oral hygiene instruction before repeating the above. The interval between appointments may be extended as cooperation is improved.

4.3.7 Advice to patients

The advice that should be given to patients has recently been reviewed in the light of the experimental evidence available.[7] The advice may be summarized as follows:

Frequency of brushing

Brush twice a day with a fluoride toothpaste.

Fluoride concentration

The choice of fluoride concentration should be based on the age and perceived caries risk of the individual and their exposure to other fluoride sources.

- A toothpaste containing 1100–1450 ppm of fluoride is appropriate for children over 7 years and adults. Children under 7 years of age should also use this paste unless they are low caries risk and living in an area where there is fluoride in the water, when a low fluoride concentration (<600 ppm) may be chosen.
- For children under 7 years, a parent should apply a small amount of paste (a pea-sized lump or smear) to the toothbrush to avoid fluorosis (see Chapter 6, page 115).
- A high-fluoride toothpaste (in UK this contains 2800 ppm fluoride) is appropriate for adults at high risk of caries. This cannot be purchased over the counter in the UK and must be prescribed by a dentist.

Toothpaste use in children

- Parents and carers should begin brushing once the primary teeth have started to erupt.
- Children under 7 years of age should be supervised. Only a pea-sized amount or smear of toothpaste should be used.
- Parents or carers should 'finish off' the brushing, paying particular attention to the occlusal surfaces of erupting teeth.

Rinsing behaviour

Discourage rinsing with large volumes of water. It is better to wet the brush, clean excess paste with this, and spit. The message is 'spit, don't rinse'. Encourage young children to spit out excess toothpaste rather than swallow it, to prevent fluorosis (see Chapter 6, page 115).

When to brush

Brush last thing at night, so that the remains of the paste remain in the mouth when asleep because salivary flow is reduced. Brush on one other occasion e.g. on rising, before breakfast. Where breakfast includes fruit juices or grapefruit teeth should not be brushed immediately afterwards to avoid creating sensitivity on any exposed areas of dentine.

Type of fluoride

Check the patient has selected a toothpaste containing fluoride. Toothpastes containing sodium fluoride, sodium monofluorophosphate, or stannous fluoride are clinically effective.

4.4 CHLORHEXIDINE: A CHEMICAL AGENT FOR PLAQUE CONTROL

Regular daily mechanical removal of plaque by the patient is the established method of plaque control, and sufficiently motivated individuals reach a high level of proficiency. However, for some others, effective removal of plaque by mechanical means may not be possible.

Physically and mentally handicapped individuals may have to rely on others for their oral hygiene. It is also painful to use a toothbrush when acute inflammation is present. Consequently, a great deal of research has been directed towards the use of chemical agents which may inhibit or suppress the deposition of plaque.

If it is believed that all plaque bacteria are potentially cariogenic, then the ideal agent must be capable of complete inhibition of plaque and must be used continuously. However, this ideal agent does not exist. Fortunately, elimination of specific microorganisms, for instance mutans streptococci, may 'throw a spanner' in the bacterial ecology and have a useful role to play in caries control. Nevertheless, any chemical agent would have to satisfy the stringent safety requirements for use in the mouth. In particular, it should not induce the emergence of resistant strains of microorganisms nor produce unwelcome side effects.

Of all the chemical agents for plaque control, chlorhexidine is the most effective and is used as the 'gold standard' to which any new agent is compared. Consequently, it will be covered in detail.

4.4.1 Mechanism of action, dosage, and delivery

Chlorhexidine is an antiseptic belonging to the chemical group of compounds called bisbiguanides which are bactericidal and fungicidal. It has a broad spectrum of activity against Gram-positive and Gram-negative organisms as well as yeasts. The chlorhexidine molecule is cationic, which means it is positively charged, and it is therefore attracted to bacterial cell walls, which are negatively charged. The bacterial cell wall is then irreversibly damaged, with subsequent precipitation of its cytoplasmic components, resulting in cell death. Because of their positive charge cationic antiseptics, when used in the mouth, adsorb to dental tissues, to the acidic proteins covering the teeth and oral mucosa, and to the proteins in saliva. It is the adsorbed antiseptic on the tooth surface that exerts the bactericidal action against organisms attempting to colonize. The success of an antiseptic as a plaque inhibitor depends not only on its antibacterial properties but also on the rate at which it is released from the tooth surface.

The plaque-inhibiting properties of a chlorhexidine **mouthrinse** were first demonstrated by Löe and Schiött.[8] They showed that, in a group of dental students, by rinsing for 1 minute twice a day with 10 ml of a 0.2% solution of chlorhexidine, plaque deposition and gingivitis could be almost entirely prevented in the absence of oral hygiene. However, in subsequent experiments on unselected subjects, although chlorhexidine was still very effective, its limitations were highlighted. It did not totally inhibit plaque in the average patient. The presence of calculus, overhanging or defective restorations, and periodontal pockets >3 mm reduced its efficacy since these factors would hamper access of the solution to vulnerable sites. Consequently, its effect is greatly enhanced by supra- and subgingival scaling and correction of defective restorations.

Since the original studies using 10 ml of a 0.2% solution as a mouthrinse, various vehicles have been used to deliver the chlorhexidine to the tooth surface. The application of 2–5 ml of a solution at the same concentration but in a **spray** has been tested with good results on a group of handicapped children. This method of delivery has been shown to be very acceptable and is therefore very useful to enable such patients to reach acceptable levels of oral cleanliness. It is also a convenient method of maintaining a clean mouth for debilitated patients or for patients with fixed oral splints. Chlorhexidine is also available in the form of a **gel** at a concentration of 1%. This can be used on a toothbrush or in custom-made vinyl applicator trays (see Figure 7.2, p. 138).

Chlorhexidine has also been incorporated into **chewing gum**. When this gum was tested in elderly patients living in residential care it was found to be both beneficial and well accepted in those who could chew. The chewing stimulated salivary flow, which was particularly helpful since many of this population have drug-induced dry mouth. The use of the chlorhexidine-containing chewing gum produced significant clinical improvements in the oral health of the frail elderly people, reducing denture debris, denture stomatitis and angular cheilitis.[9]

4.4.2 Side effects

Staining

The most conspicuous side effect is the development of a yellow or brown stain on the teeth and tongue and on the margins of anterior restorations. Staining around these restorations can be prevented if they are coated with Vaseline before rinsing. The stain is caused by the interaction of chlorhexidine with certain constituents of the diet. It is more severe following mouthrinses and in the absence of toothbrushing, and is increased by excessive intake of tea, coffee, and red wine. Professional cleaning is required to remove it, but when it accumulates around the margins of defective restorations it is impossible to remove. This limits the long-term use of chlorhexidine.

Taste

Chlorhexidine has a bitter taste and there is a general dulling of taste sensation for a few minutes to several hours after rinsing, depending on the individual. The bitter taste has been masked quite successfully by flavouring agents.

Parotid gland swelling

A few cases of unilateral or bilateral swelling of the parotid glands have been reported. However, they were all reversible when rinsing was discontinued.

Desquamation of oral mucosa

There may be individual variation in the tolerance level of the oral mucosa to chlorhexidine. Consequently, a few cases of painful desquamatous lesions have been reported. All cases resolved when rinsing was discontinued or when the mouthwash was diluted 1 : 1 with water. When the mouthrinse is prescribed for patients whose oral mucosa is compromised due to desquamation or ulceration, they should be advised to add water to the original 10 ml dose until it no longer causes stinging. It is also important to instruct the patient to use the total diluted volume to achieve maximum plaque inhibition.

Long-term effects

The effects of 2 years' regular use of chlorhexidine have been studied. There were no untoward lasting consequences. There is a slight change in the balance of oral flora in favour of the organisms that are less sensitive to it, but this returns to normal after 3 months. Gingival biopsies taken 18 months after daily use by human subjects showed no histological abnormalities.

4.4.3 The use of chlorhexidine in the control of caries

Patients with greatly reduced salivary flow, who are consequently very much 'at risk' to caries, may benefit from the prophylactic use of chlorhexidine in conjunction with fluoride (see sections 7.4.3 and 7.4.4). Chlorhexidine should never be regarded as a substitute for mechanical plaque control but as an added measure in cases where caries is uncontrolled.

Further reading and references

1. Fejerskov, O. and Kidd, E. A. M. (eds) (2003) *Dental caries*. Ch.11: The role of oral hygiene. Blackwell Munksgaard, Oxford.
2. Fehr, F. R. von der, Löe, H. and Theilade, E. (1970) Experimental caries in man. *Caries Res.*, **4**, 131–148.
3. Marinho, V. C. C., Higgins, J. P. T., Sheiham, A., and Logon, S. (2003) Fluoride toothpastes for preventing caries in children and adolescents. (Cochrane Review). *Cochrane Library, Issue 1*. Software Update, Oxford.
4. Axelsson, P. and Lindhe, J. (1974) The effect of a preventive programme on dental plaque, gingivitis and caries in schoolchildren. Results after one and two years. *J. Clin Periodontol.*, **1**, 126–138.
5. Heanue, M., Deacon, S. A. A., and Deery, C. *et al.* (2003) Manual versus powered toothbrushing for oral health. (Cochrane Review). *Cochrane Library, Issue 1*. Software Update, Oxford.
6. Clarkson, J. E., Ellwood, R. P., and Chandler, R. E. (1993) A comprehensive summary of fluoride dentifrice caries clinical trials. *Am. J. Dent.*, **6**(Spec. Iss.), S59–106.
7. Davies, R. M., Davies, G. M., and Ellwood, R. P. (2003) Prevention. Part 4: Toothbrushing: What advice should be given to patients? *Br. Dent. J.*, **195**, 135–141.
8. Löe, H. and Schiött, C. R. (1970) The effect of mouthrinses and topical applications of chlorhexidine on the development of dental plaque and gingivitis in man. *J. Periodont. Res.*, Suppl. no. 12, **8**, 5–99.
9. Simons, D., Brailsford, S. R., Kidd, E. A. M., and Beighton, D. (2002) The use of medicated chewing gums and oral health in frail elderly people: a one-year clinical trial. *J. Am. Geriatric Soc.*, **50**, 1348–1353.

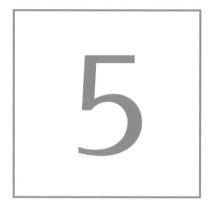

Diet and caries

5.1   ACID PRODUCTION IN DENTAL PLAQUE

Fermentable carbohydrate and a cariogenic plaque need to be present on a tooth surface for acid to form. The acid is produced by bacterial metabolism of the carbohydrate substrate. The process is well illustrated by the Stephan curves shown in Figure 1.6 (page 17). This figure illustrates that the resting pH attained can vary with the tooth surface under test. Thus plaque within active occlusal carious cavities has a lower resting pH value than plaque on inactive occlusal carious lesions or sound surfaces. Similarly, after the sucrose rinse, the plaque within an active cavity shows the greatest fall in pH and remains low for longest. This demonstrates the relevance of operative dentistry in caries control and will be referred to again in Chapter 9.

Thus a single sucrose rinse, lasting a matter of seconds, can cause de-mineralization lasting between 20 minutes and several hours. Many factors determine the shape of the Stephan curve. The gradual return of pH to base-line values is a result of acids diffusing out of the plaque. In addition, buffers in the plaque and salivary film exert a neutralizing effect. Saliva is very important in countering pH drops, and this is one reason why people with dry mouths are at high risk of active caries. It also explains how stimulation of saliva can help to counteract a fall in pH.

There has been a vast amount of experimental work linking fermentable carbohydrate and dental caries.[1,2] This work has proved that sugar is the most important dietary item in caries aetiology. Thus dietary advice has an important role in the management of the carious process, in conjunction with oral hygiene and use of fluoride.

5.2   SOME EVIDENCE LINKING DIET AND CARIES

5.2.1   Epidemiological evidence

The consumption of sugar in substantial amounts is a recent trend in many areas of the world. Evidence linking sugar and caries has come from communities whose caries status has been recorded before and after an increase in the availability of sugar. One of the best known examples is the dental status of the inhabitants of Tristan da Cuhna, a remote rocky island in the South Atlantic. Their dental state was excellent in the 1930s when their diet comprised potatoes and other vegetables, meat, and fish. However, after 1940, there was a sharp increase in the consumption of imported sugary foods and a commensurate increase in caries.

The severe dietary restrictions in many countries during World War II were accompanied by a decrease in dental caries. The teeth which had already erupted showed the same reduced caries score as the developing teeth, and the improvement was therefore due to a local dietary effect rather than a systemic nutritional one.

Epidemiological studies on other groups of people eating low amounts of sugar have also yielded interesting results. In 1942 an eccentric, wealthy Australian businessman transformed a spacious country mansion, Hopewood House, into a home for young children of low socio-economic background. When the children were 12 years old they could move to other accommodation but remained associated with the house. Since this entrepreneur attributed his own improvement in health to a drastic change in dietary habits, he stipulated that the children should be raised on a natural diet excluding refined carbohydrates. The dental surveys revealed a very low prevalence and severity of dental caries, much lower than in children of the same age and socioeconomic background attending ordinary state schools in New South Wales. However, after 12 years of age, when close supervision ended, their caries rate became virtually the same as that in the children in the state schools. This indicates that the diet eaten up to the age of 12 years did not confer any subsequent protection.

Another piece of evidence linking diet and caries concerns the rare hereditary disease fructose intolerance, which is caused by an inborn error of metabolism. Patients with this disease lack a certain liver enzyme, and ingestion of foods containing fructose or sucrose causes severe nausea. Consequently they avoid these foods. The caries experience of these patients is very low, indicating that a group of people who are not able to tolerate many sugary foods are unlikely to develop much caries.

5.2.2   Interventional human clinical studies

An interventional study is one that measures the effects of altering, or intervening, in the study conditions in some way. In the dental field perhaps the most famous of all human clinical studies was begun in 1939 when the Swedish Government requested an investigation into what measures should be taken to reduce the frequency of the most common dental disease in Sweden. This led to a study on the relationship between diet and dental caries which was carried out at the Vipeholm Hospital, an institution for mentally handicapped individuals. The hospital, with its large number of permanent patients, provided an opportunity for a longitudinal study under well-controlled conditions. A comparable study on human subjects will probably never be repeated as it would now be regarded as unethical to alter diets experimentally in directions likely to increase caries.

The patients were divided into one control and six experimental groups. Four meals were eaten daily and for one year patients received a diet relatively low in sugar with no sugar between meals. During this time the number of new carious lesions was assessed and found to be very low. Subsequently, the effect on caries of dietary changes involving the addition of large sucrose supplements in sticky or non-sticky form, either with or between meals, was assessed.

The control group, who continued with the basic diet, showed little increase in caries throughout the study. In the experimental groups the diet was supplemented by sucrose drinks or sucrose in bread or chocolate or caramels, or 8 toffees or 24 toffees per day. There was a marked increase in caries in all groups except when the sucrose drink was taken at meal times. The risk of sugar increasing the caries activity was greatest if the sugar was taken between meals, in a sticky form. Indeed, in the 24-toffee groups, when the toffees were eaten between meals, the increase in caries was so great that the sugar supplement was withdrawn. This resulted in a fall in caries increment.

Dentists now base much of their dietary advice on the results of this study, stressing that the frequency of sugar intake should be reduced to confine sugar to meal times as far as possible. They advise against sticky, sweet foods and maintain that the rate of development of new disease will fall if this dietary advice is followed.

Another large-scale and important experiment on caries in humans was carried out in Turku, Finland, the aim being to compare the cariogenicity of sucrose, fructose, and xylitol. Xylitol is a sugar alcohol which is sweet but is not metabolized to acid by plaque microorganisms. The results of the study showed that both sucrose and fructose were cariogenic, but the almost total substitution of sucrose by xylitol resulted in a substantial reduction in caries incidence. This introduces the concept that it may be possible to substitute sucrose by substances which will impart sweetness but are not cariogenic, which is covered in more detail in section 5.11.2.

5.2.3   Non-interventional human studies

A non-interventional study relies on measurement alone, without any active intervention in the study conditions. There have been a number of cross-sectional surveys of populations in which investigators have attempted to relate dietary habits to the prevalence of caries. Information about dietary habits is gathered by questionnaires and the caries data by clinical examination to obtain the DMF data. However, the latter represents a lifetime's caries experience and this may not correspond to 'snapshot' dietary diaries. Although some studies showed significant relationships between the amount and frequency of sugar intake and caries status, others did not.

Two longitudinal (two- and three-year) studies of adolescent schoolchildren living in communities with minimal fluoride in the drinking water were conducted in Northumberland, UK,[3] and Michigan, USA.[4] Dietary histories were recorded and related to the caries that developed over the same time period. The correlations between the caries increments and dietary factors were positive but low. However, when the caries increments of children with the highest and lowest sugar intakes were compared, obvious differences emerged.

The relative cariogenicity of starch and sugars was evaluated in a 2-year longitudinal dietary study of English schoolchildren that monitored both dietary intake and caries increment. When carbohydrate intake was examined, a lower mean caries increment was found for the high starch/low sugars group compared with the low starch/high sugars group.[5]

5.2.4   Animal experiments

The most commonly used animal in caries experiments is the rat, but hamsters, mice and monkeys have also been used. One of the most important animal experiments was reported in 1954, when a system for rearing rats under germ-free conditions was devised. When these rats, who had no bacteria in their mouths, were fed a cariogenic diet, caries did not develop. This showed that a cariogenic oral microflora is essential for the development of dental caries.

Subsequently, the importance of the local effect of diet in the mouth was demonstrated when animals fed a cariogenic diet via a stomach tube did not develop the disease. Rat experiments have also confirmed the positive correlation between frequency of sugar intake and caries severity.

Animal experiments are commonly used to compare the cariogenicity of foods. Such work has shown that sucrose, glucose, fructose, galactose, lactose, and maltose are all cariogenic in varying degrees, with sucrose being the most cariogenic.

Animal experiments on the cariogenicity of starch have yielded conflicting results, showing starch products with a cariogenicity ranging from very low to comparable to that of glucose! Heating at temperatures used in cooking and baking causes a partial degradation of starch, so it is possible that cooked starch may be capable of fermentation to acid in the mouth.

5.3   FREQUENCY OR AMOUNT OF SUGARS

Both frequency and amount of sugars are associated with dental caries. In the UK and many developed countries the public health message is to reduce the amount of sugars consumed. However, at the level of the individual patient, it is more practical to advise limiting frequency of intake. Since frequency and amount of sugar consumed are closely associated, efforts to reduce frequency are also likely to reduce the quantity consumed.

5.4   HAS FLUORIDE INFLUENCED THE RELATIONSHIP BETWEEN SUGAR AND CARIES?

The relationships between childhood caries experience and sucrose availability over 50 years in children in England and Wales are illustrated graphically in Figure 5.1.[6] This graph is taken from an interesting paper in which it was concluded that the most likely explanation for the pattern of disease observed was the increase and then reduction in sugar challenge to the population. However, from the beginning of the 1970s this relationship was influenced by the preventive effect of fluoride in toothpaste. It was suggested that this accounted for the very steep decline in caries in children from this time.

Fluoride has had a marked effect on caries reduction but it has not eliminated the ubiquitous, natural process that is caries. In this process the bacteria in the biofilm metabolize sugar to produce acid. Fluoride has probably increased the safe margin of sugar intake but, despite the widespread use of fluoride, the frequency and amount of sugars intake remain important determinants of caries levels. A systematic review of the evidence for an association between sugar intake and dental caries in modern society has concluded that restriction of sugar consumption still has a role to play in caries prevention, but on a community level this role is not as vital as it was in the pre-fluoride era.[7]

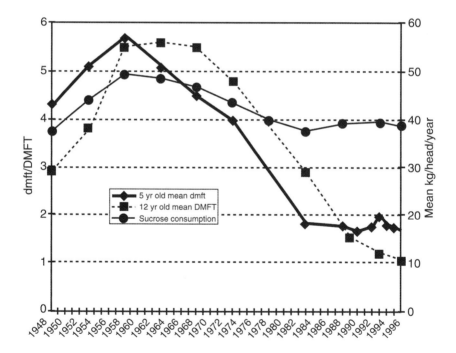

Figure 5.1. Dental caries experience of 5-year-old (dmft) and 12-year-old children (DMFT) in England (1948–1968) and England and Wales (1973–1997), and sucrose available for consumption (kg/head per year) in the United Kingdom (1948–1998) (Downer, M. C. (1999). Caries experience and sucrose availability: an analysis of the relationship in the United Kingdom over fifty years. *Community Dental Health.* **16**,18–21.) Reproduced by courtesy of the Editor of *Community Dental Health.*

5.5   CLASSIFICATION OF SUGARS FOR DENTAL HEALTH PURPOSES[8]

Sugars integrated into the cellular structure of food (e.g. in fruit) are called **intrinsic sugars**. Sugars present in a free form (e.g. table sugar) or added to food (e.g. sweets, biscuits) are called **extrinsic sugars**. These may be more readily available for metabolism by the oral bacteria and are therefore potentially more cariogenic.

Milk contains lactose but is not generally regarded as cariogenic. Cheese and yoghurts, without added sugars, may also be considered safe for teeth. Thus the most damaging sugars for dental health are **non-milk extrinsic sugars** (NMES).

5.6   RECOMMENDED AND CURRENT LEVELS OF SUGAR INTAKE[8]

The recommended intake of non-milk extrinsic sugars is a maximum of 60 g/day, which is about 10% of daily energy intake. However, the latest National Diet and Nutrition Survey of young people aged 4–18 years showed mean NMES intakes at 85 g/day in boys and 69 g/day in girls.[9] The main source of these sugars was soft drinks and confectionery. These tend to be consumed between meals and contribute to obesity. Dietary advice from the dentist is a part of an overall healthy diet promotion message.

5.7   STARCH, FRUIT, AND FRUIT SUGARS[8]

Raw starch (e.g. raw vegetables) is of low cariogenicity. However, cooked and highly refined starch (e.g. crisps) can cause decay, and combinations of cooked starch and sucrose (e.g. cakes, biscuits, sugared breakfast cereals) can be highly cariogenic.

Current dietary advice recommends at least five portions of fruit and vegetables per day. Fruit contains sugars (fructose, sucrose, and glucose) but fresh fruits appear to be of low cariogenicity. However, the same cannot be said for fruit juice. The juicing process releases the sugars from the whole fruit, and these drinks are potentially cariogenic. Dried fruit is also cariogenic. These products are sticky, tending to adhere to teeth, and the drying process releases some of the intrinsic sugars.

5.8   CULTURAL AND SOCIAL PRESSURES

Vast capital sums are invested in the sugar industry and related industries manufacturing soft drinks and confectionery. Large sums of money are also spent advertising sugar products, and the public are constantly exhorted to purchase sweet food products which they are told provide instant energy.

Sweets are often placed next to check-outs in supermarkets and school tuck shops, and chocolate-bearing grannies flourish. In addition, many foods which are not generally thought of as cariogenic contain significant amounts of sucrose (sometimes called 'hidden sugar'), for example, tomato soup, mustard, tomato sauce, frozen pears, tinned pasta, breakfast cereals, fruit yoghurts, many savoury baby foods, and rusks.

5.9 GROUPS AT PARTICULAR RISK OF CARIES IN RELATION TO DIET[2]

Some people, with a particular behaviour, medical problem, or relevant biological factor are of particular risk to caries because of dietary factors. Since caries is a multifactorial disease the relationship is not simple. It cannot be said that all in a particular group will have a problem with caries, but these groups are worth listing, because they should at least sound 'warning bells' in the dentist's mind.

- infants and toddlers with prolonged breast-feeding on demand
- infants and toddlers provided with a feeding bottle at bedtime, or bottle suspended in the cot for use during the night, with a sugar-containing liquid
- people with an increased frequency of eating because of a medical problem, e.g. gastrointestinal disease, eating disorders, uncontrolled diabetes
- those with an increased carbohydrate intake due to a medical problem, e.g. Crohn's disease, chronic renal failure, other chronic illness, malnutrition, or failure to thrive
- those with reduced salivary secretion leading to a prolonged clearance rate of sugars and a Stephan curve that takes longer than usual to return to a neutral pH, e.g. those on medications causing reduced salivary flow, Sjögren's syndrome, irradiation in the region of the salivary glands
- athletes taking sugar-containing sport supplement drinks
- workers subject to occupational hazards such as food sampling, those working in the confectionery and bakery industry and those on a monotonous job such as a night shift
- drug abusers who have a craving for sugar and a prolonged clearance rate as a result of reduced salivary secretion
- people, of any age, on long term and/or multiple medications. Are these sugars-based and/or do they cause a dry mouth?

5.10 DIET ANALYSIS

The practical problems of diet analysis and advice in the caries-prone patient should be tackled systematically. Initially, the patient's current diet should be determined because this baseline information is needed if sensible advice is to be given. Dietary analysis should be carried out on all patients with a high caries activity and in those with an unusual caries pattern.

There are two principal techniques for determining food intake. One is to record the dietary intake during the preceding 24 hours, the so-called **24-hour recall** system. This involves careful history taking and relies on the patient's memory and honesty. The other method is to obtain a **3–4 day written diet record**, the patient recording food and liquid intake as it is consumed. This relies on the patient's full cooperation as well as honesty.

Both forms of diet recording suffer from the disadvantage that the record may not be representative of the diet consumed over a much longer time, although it is this which is likely to have been responsible for the caries and restoration status with which the patient presents. Thus, a diet history is an unscientific tool and must be interpreted with caution.

5.10.1 Recording the diet

In the author's unit, we use a diet sheet as shown in Figure 5.2. When we give this to patients we explain that their help is needed to find the cause of their dental decay. The cause is related to what they eat and drink, and for this reason it is necessary for them to record everything eaten and drunk over a

Diet Analysis

	THURSDAY		FRIDAY		SATURDAY		SUNDAY	
	Time	Item	Time	Item	Time	Item	Time	Item
BEFORE BREAKFAST								
Breakfast								
MORNING								
Mid-day meal								
AFTERNOON								
Evening meal								
EVENING and NIGHT								

Figure 5.2. A form on which a patient may record diet over a 4-day period. This has been designed to highlight the between-meal snack, thus facilitating patient education when the sheet is completed and returned. On the reverse side of the diet sheet there are simple instructions explaining how it should be filled in.

4-day period, together with the time of eating. (In addition, any medication should be entered.) They are requested to keep the diet sheet with them and fill it in at the time, to avoid missing anything. Quantities of food consumed are not specifically requested, but it should be stressed that nothing should be changed because a record is being kept. Dentist and patient are partners in the investigation and the object of the exercise is to help, not to condemn.

Although this strategy is useful for many patients, it may be inappropriate for others. Sometimes variable dietary habits will mean that the 4-day record is inappropriate or even misleading. Shift workers may have different dietary habits from week to week, as may those whose work necessitates frequent trips abroad. 'Bingers' will be unwilling to commit their usual dietary pattern to paper. A medical history may reveal unstable health conditions such as intermittent ulcer problems, and thus a 4-day record may be inappropriate. However, if the patient understands the purpose of the record, they may suggest how best it is kept. For instance, a shift worker may record 2 days on duty and 2 days off. Those with a medical history may record typical days when they are 'well' and other days when they are 'ill'. Finally it must be appreciated that a patient may not always tell the truth, although if they know what to lie about, progress has been made!

5.10.2   Analysis of the dietary record

Once the patient returns the completed sheet, dentist and patient can begin to look at it together. A highlighter pen is useful to mark items containing sugar. If the dentist encourages the patient to identify these, it will become apparent whether the patient realizes which items are sweet.

The relevance of sugar and the role of bacterial plaque should be explained, and then the number of sugar attacks can be counted and this number recorded at the top of each day. This gives the dentist the opportunity to explain the relevance of frequency of sugar attacks. The amount of time the plaque remains acid and capable of causing demineralization varies depending on such factors as the consistency of the food, salivary flow, salivary clearance rates, and the activity of the carious lesion.

However, these complex and important scientific deliberations will be lost on the patient who needs a simple (but scientifically simplistic) message. It would not be unreasonable to suggest that after a sugar attack the plaque is likely to remain acid for 1 hour, thus 8 attacks would equal 8 hours of acid plaque.

Special note is taken of:
- the main meals, to see whether they are sufficiently substantial—this is important to prevent the patient craving food between meals
- the between-meal snacks. Are they cariogenic?
- any medication, particularly if it is based on a sucrose syrup or if it is likely to cause dry mouth or thirst

- the number and type of between-meal drinks. Are these cariogenic?
- the consistency of any between-meal snacks. Are they sticky and therefore take a long time to clear from the mouth?
- the use of sucrose-containing chewing gum or any sweet that takes a long time to dissolve in the mouth
- any sugary bedtime snacks or drinks.

Figures 5.3–5.5 show examples of diet analysis sheets. Figure 5.3 is one day from a diet sheet kept by a 24-year-old mechanical engineer referred to a consultant from a practitioner because of a high caries rate. The patient was an intelligent young man, concerned about his teeth and grateful for all his dentist was doing for him. The mouth was clean and well restored but white spot lesions were developing around the margins of restorations and the dentist's radiographs, taken at yearly intervals, showed that approximal enamel lesions were progressing into dentine. The diet sheet shows 10 separate sugar attacks, including a sugary drink just before bed. The patient ate frequently and used the term 'grazing' to describe his eating habits. All drinks were cariogenic and the main meals were inadequate because he ate as he worked.

DIET ANALYSIS

		THURSDAY
	Time	10 attacks Item 1 pre-bed
BEFORE BREAK-FAST	7.15	1 pint skimmed milk milk shake
Breakfast	8.30	Black coffee + Sugar
MORNING	10.00 / 12.00	White coffee + Sugar / 2 cheese rolls / Bag Crisps, Cake / Twix / White coffee + Sugar
Mid-day Meal	13.30	2 cheese rolls / Cake / 1 mint / Apple
AFTER-NOON	15.30 / 17.00	White coffee + Sugar / Tea + Sugar / 4 Biscuits
Evening Meal	19.30	Pizza / Ribena / Ice Cream
EVENING	21.30 / 22.30	Glass of coke / Glass of coke

Figure 5.3. One day in the initial diet sheet of a 24-year-old mechanical engineer.

DIET ANALYSIS (See notes on other side) ✳ = 2 spoons of sugar.

	THURSDAY		FRIDAY		SATURDAY		SUNDAY	
	Time	Item	Time	Item	Time	Item	Time	Item
BEFORE BREAKFAST	7.45	Tea ✳	7.00	Tea ✳	7.00	Tea ✳		
Breakfast	9.00	Coffee ✳	8.45	Coffee ✳	10.00	Tea ✳ 2 pieces of toast		
MORNING	10.00	Coffee ✳ Roll and butter	9.30	Coffee ✳	11.00	Coffee ✳	10.45	Tea ✳
	10.45	Coffee ✳	10.45	Roll and butter Coffee ✳	12.00	Coffee ✳	11.30	Tea ✳
			11.45	Coffee ✳				
Mid–day Meal	12.30	Coffee ✳	1.45	Cheese & onion Sandwich ½ Lager	1.0	Coffee ✳ 1. muesli biscuit	2.0	Beef: roast potatoes Carrots : greens fresh pear Tea ✳
	1.30	Coffee ✳						
AFTERNOON	2.30	Coffee ✳	2.30	Coffee ✳	3.00	Tea ✳		
	3.45	Coffee ✳	3.15	Coffee ✳	4.15	Tea ✳	3.30	Tea ✳
	4.15	Coffee ✳	4.00	Coffee ✳				
			5.00	Coffee ✳				
Evening Meal	7.30	Country hash Tea ✳	9.00	Lasagne Tea ✳	7.00	Spare Ribs, Rice Tea ✳	5.00	Tea ✳
							6.30	Coffee ✳
EVENING & NIGHT	9.00	2 muesli biscuits	10.00	Tea ✳	9.30	Tea ✳	8.00	Coffee ✳
		Tea ✳	11.15	Tea ✳ 2 biscuits	11.00	Tea ✳	10.00	Cheese & biscuit Tea ✳
	10.30	Pear						

Figure 5.4. A diet sheet completed by a middle-aged secretary with a very high incidence of caries. This lady returned to the surgery saying that she now realized that drinking frequent cups of sweetened tea and coffee was the likely cause of her caries.

The diet sheet in Figure 5.4 is from a middle-aged secretary with a high incidence of caries. This patient returned to the surgery after having kept the record, saying that she now realized the cause of the decay in her mouth. In addition, she said how surprised she was to see how little she ate at meal times.

Figure 5.5 shows one day in a remarkable diet where the patient drank regularly every 2 hours, day and night. The relevant feature of this diet sheet was that the patient was taking chlorpromazine (Largactil), an antipsychotic drug, and lithium carbonate for depression. These drugs cause dry mouth and thirst respectively (see Chapter 7); consequently the patient was continually drinking, and many of these drinks were cariogenic. Unfortunately the remains of the dentition were beyond repair and the patient is now edentulous.

5.11 DIETARY ADVICE

On the basis of the diet analysis, the clinician may be in a position to indicate to the patient which constituents of the diet may be harmful and to make some positive recommendations. Dietary advice should be tailored to the needs of the individual patient and should form part of a comprehensive pre-

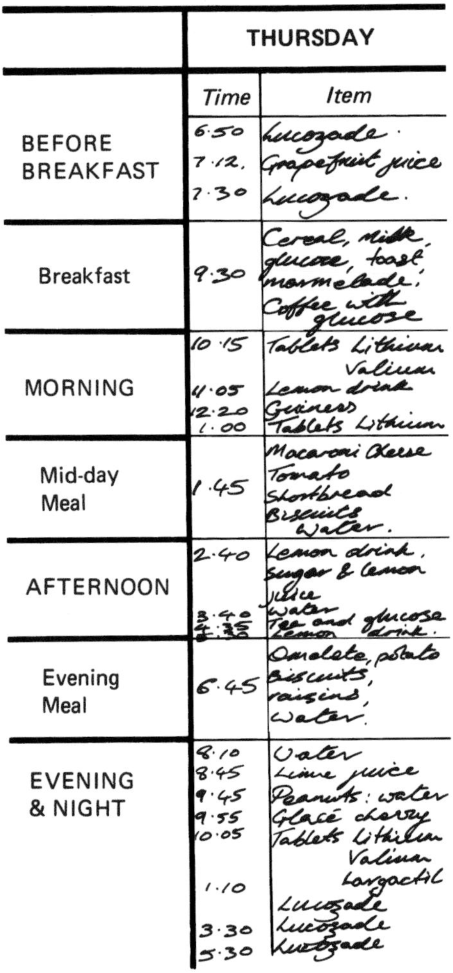

	THURSDAY	
	Time	*Item*
BEFORE BREAKFAST	6.50	Lucozade
	7.12.	Grapefruit juice
	7.30	Lucozade.
Breakfast	9.30	Cereal, milk, glucose, toast, marmelade, Coffee with glucose
MORNING	10.15	Tablets Lithium Valium
	11.05	Lemon drink
	12.20	Guiness
	1.00	Tablets Lithium
Mid-day Meal	1.45	Macaroni Cheese Tomato Shortbread Biscuits Water.
AFTERNOON	2.40	Lemon drink, sugar & lemon juice
	3.40	water and glucose
	4.35	Tea and lemon drink.
Evening Meal	6.45	Omelete, potato Biscuits, raisins, water.
EVENING & NIGHT	8.10	Water
	8.45	Lime juice
	9.45	Peanuts: water
	9.55	Glacé cherry
	10.05	Tablets Lithium Valium Largactil
	1.10	Lucozade
	3.30	Lucozade
	5.30	Lucozade

Figure 5.5. One day from an unusual diet sheet kept by a patient who was thirsty because of her medication and consequently drank regularly. Unfortunately most of the drinks were cariogenic.

ventive programme consisting of oral hygiene instructions, the use of topical fluoride preparations, and operative dentistry to facilitate plaque control.

5.11.1 General advice

Dietary advice provided by dental health professions should correspond to the general nutritional recommendations for good health (see upper box overleaf).

Dietary advice must be practical, setting realistic goals (see section 8.5.10). It is impossible to expect patients to cut sugar completely out of the diet, but it is feasible to reduce the total amount of sugar consumed, and to restrict sugar intake mainly to meal times.

NUTRITIONAL RECOMMENDATIONS FOR GOOD HEALTH[10]

- Enjoy your food
- Eat a variety of different foods
- Eat the right amount to be a healthy weight
- Eat plenty of foods rich in starch and fibre
- Eat plenty of fruit and vegetables
- Don't eat too many foods that contain a lot of fat
- Don't have sugary foods and drinks too often
- If you drink alcohol, drink sensibly

FOODS AND DRINKS WITH LOW POTENTIAL FOR DENTAL CARIES

- Bread (sandwiches, toast, crumpets, pitta bread).
- Pasta, rice, starchy staple foods
- Cheese
- Fibrous foods (e.g. raw vegetables)
- Low sugar breakfast cereals (e.g. shredded wheat)
- Fresh fruit (whole and not juices)
- Peanuts (not for children under 5 years)
- Sugar-free chewing gum
- Sugar-free confectionery
- Water
- Milk
- Sugar-free drinks
- Tea and coffee (unsweetened)

Sugary foods or drinks between meals are particularly harmful and should be avoided in the caries-prone patient. Fruit, peanuts, or cheese may be acceptable alternatives, although peanuts should not be given to children under 5 years as there is a real risk of death due to asphyxiation following inhalation of a single nut. The bed-time snack or drink is particularly important, since salivary flow is virtually absent at night and plaque pH may remain low for many hours.

It is neither necessary nor practical to stop children eating sweets altogether. However, it is not unreasonable to suggest that they are restricted to one day a week. In any case, children should be encouraged to eat a balanced meal before any sweets are given. If sweets are eaten, they will do least damage as part of a main meal. Granny's advice of 'Don't eat them all at once', as she hands over the chocolates, could be disastrous for dental health.

Adults should also be advised not to eat sugary snacks between meals, but if sugary snacks are cut out of the diet the patient may be hungry and thus a list of snack-foods and drinks with a low potential for dental caries (see lower box opposite) is useful so that the patient may suggest a suitable alternative. However, it is often sweetened drinks that are the problem, and here sugar substitutes can be very helpful.

5.11.2   Sugar substitutes

There is increasing interest in the use of sweetening agents which confer sweetness but are safer for teeth. They are useful because many people have a sweet tooth and thus when sugar substitutes are used to replace sugars in foods that are frequently consumed, such as sweet snacks, drinks, and liquid medicines, they will have dental benefits. These products may be divided into two categories: those which have no calorific value (non-nutritive or intense sweeteners) and those which have a calorific value (nutritive or bulk sweeteners). The non-sugar sweeteners currently permitted in the UK are shown in Table 5.1, together with a list of sugars or substances containing sugar. This list should be useful when helping a patient to examine food labels to see if the constituents are potentially cariogenic.

Table 5.1 Sweeteners

| | Sugar substitutes | |
Sugar or sugar containing	Non-nutritive	Nutritive
Sucrose	Saccharin	Sorbitol
Glucose	Acesulfame-K	Mannitol
Glucose syrup	Aspartame	Xylitol
Fructose	Thaumatin	Maltitol
Sorbose		Hydrogenated
Lactose		glucose syrup
Maltose		(Lycasin)
Dextrose		Isomalt (Palatinit)
Honey		
Corn syrup		
Invert sugar syrup		
Molasses		
Treacle		

Non-nutritive sweeteners

These are sometimes called **intense sweeteners** because they have a sweetness many times that of sucrose. These substances impart sweetness but furnish no calories. They are safe for teeth because they cannot act as an energy source for dental plaque microorganisms and acid cannot be derived from them.

The three non-nutritive sweeteners readily available in the UK are saccharin, acesulfame-K, and aspartame. They are produced in both tablet and granule form, but the granule form is best avoided because the bulking agent is maltodextrin, which may be cariogenic. Saccharin was discovered more than a century ago and has been used as a sweetener in foods and drinks for over 80 years. It is 300 times as sweet as sugar weight for weight but suffers the disadvantage of a bitter, metallic aftertaste which some consumers find unacceptable. For some years its safety was debated because bladder tumours were found in male rats fed on exceptionally high doses of saccharin. However, it has been found to be safe, even at very high levels, for human consumption.

Acesulfame-K is chemically related to saccharin but has an improved aftertaste. Aspartame (trade names Canderel, NutraSweet) is a slightly different product containing two amino acids. Its taste is regarded as the closest to that of sucrose, with no bitterness.

Ideally these various sweeteners should be kept in the surgery so that tea or coffee can be made sweetened with these various alternatives and the patient invited to taste and rank them for acceptability (see section 8.5.9). It is a subjective impression that patients vary in what they find acceptable, and there are patients (and dental students) who cannot distinguish the sugar substitute from sugar!

These artificial sweeteners are also used in the manufacture of several drinks and, from a caries point of view, substitution of the artificially sweetened beverage may be helpful. However, it must be remembered that such drinks, although not cariogenic, are very acidic and may cause erosion if consumed frequently.

Nutritive sweeteners

The nutritive sweeteners are sugar alcohols; the most useful are sorbitol and xylitol. Other polyols used as bulk sweeteners in confectionary products are lycasin, maltitol and mannitol. **Sorbitol** is found naturally in some fruits and berries, but for economic reasons both sorbitol and **mannitol** are prepared industrially from glucose. Sorbitol is only about half as sweet as sucrose and relatively inexpensive. It is used in chewing gum, sugar-free sweets, 'diabetic' food products, sugar-free medicines, and toothpaste. Since it is only partially absorbed from the bowel, large amounts cause a laxative effect because of osmotic transfer of water into the bowel. Sorbitol is fermented by some plaque microorganisms but at a much slower rate than sucrose. There is a suggestion that with long-term use by humans the oral microflora will adapt and start to be able to convert it to acid so that it may not be completely safe for use in patients with dry mouths. However, it is regarded as much less cariogenic than sucrose. Drinks, sweets, and chewing gum containing sorbitol are likely to be safer for teeth than their sucrose-containing counterparts.

Xylitol is a sugar alcohol obtained commercially from birch trees, coconut shells, and cotton seed hulls. It is twice as expensive to produce as sorbitol and ten times the cost of sucrose. Like sorbitol it has a laxative effect, but, unlike sorbitol it cannot be fermented by oral microorganisms. Xylitol may even have an anticaries effect. Chewing gum stimulates salivary flow and xylitol reduces the levels of mutans streptococci in the mouth. This makes it a very attractive agent to put in chewing gum as a sweetening agent where chewing may encourage salivary flow and xylitol reduce the cariogenic microflora.

Hydrogenated glucose syrup (Lycasin) is obtained by enzymatic hydrolysis of corn starch. It is potentially very confusing that hydrogenated glucose syrup is sugar-free, whereas glucose syrup is basically a solution of glucose and is cariogenic. Lycasin is the registered trade mark of hydrogenated glucose syrup and is used in confectionery and pharmaceutical products in several countries. It has less of a laxative effect than other sugar alcohols.

Isomalt (Palatinit) is a mixture of two disaccharide alcohols and is said to be particularly useful in the manufacture of sugar-free chocolate.

5.11.3   Protective foods

The consumption of some foods after sugar has been shown to raise plaque pH. Cheese is useful in this respect, and can be recommended as the last course of a meal or as a 'safe' snack. Chewing gums containing xylitol have also been shown to raise salivary pH after a sugar snack.

5.11.4   'Safe' snacks

It is really remarkably difficult to draw up a list of snacks that are safe in all respects. Although cheese is safe for teeth, its high content of saturated fat may not please cardiologists. Fruit is less cariogenic than sweets, but contains natural sugar. Dried fruits such as raisins and apricots have a high sugar content and cannot be considered as 'safe' snacks. Many fruits are very acid (lemons, sour apples, oranges, grapefruit) and excessive use of such fruits or their juices may cause acid erosion of the dental tissues. However, used in moderation, fruit is safer than sweets. Nuts are a safe snack for older children and adults.

Bread and unsweetened biscuits are relatively safe for teeth, provided they are not spread with jam or honey. Some raw vegetables such as carrots and tomatoes are 'safe' but are not to everyone's taste. A list of sugar-free snacks and drinks should be used when giving dietary advice (see lower box on p. 100). The dentist should encourage patients to suggest their own solutions to problems, then write down the advice that has been agreed in the notes in a legible form for the patient to take away. Figure 5.6 shows the list of suggestions drawn up with the 24-year-old mechanical engineer whose diet sheet is seen in Figure 5.3. At the patient's next visit this list was discussed again to see which suggestions were realistic and therefore taken on board (see section 8.5.11).

SUGGESTIONS

1. Aim 2–3 sugar attacks/day
2. Never sugar before bed
3. Coffee and tea—try no sugar
4. If coke; use <u>diet</u> variety
5. Water is safe (patient hates milk!)
6. Try savory roll to eat at work
7. Try to eat more lunch and reduce 'grazing'!
8. Eat lots in evening
9. Beer is not cariogenic!

Figure 5.6. The written suggestions for dietary change given to the 24-year-old mechanical engineer whose diet sheet is seen in Figure 5.3. Each suggestion has been discussed with the patient and agreed as 'worth a try'.

5.11.5 Advice to pregnant and nursing mothers

There is little evidence in contemporary populations that children suffer any dental abnormalities due to maternal malnutrition. Nor is there evidence to suggest there will be any significant benefit to the teeth from a pregnant woman eating additional minerals, vitamins, or fluoride. There is no apparent relationship between nutritional deficiencies during tooth formation and caries.

Breast-feeding is strongly recommended by paediatricians since there is strong evidence that the number of infections and allergic conditions such as eczema are reduced in children who are breast-fed, probably because of the antibodies present in human milk. From a cariogenic point of view, it is widely believed that breast-feeding is less harmful than bottle-feeding. This may be because breast milk contains lactose which is significantly less cariogenic than sucrose. However, very rare cases of rampant caries have been described in infants breast-feeding on true demand for up to 2 years or more. In this condition the infants suckle regularly through the day and the night, perhaps 60 times per 24-hour period, for several years.

The practice of adding sugar or honey to baby foods should be discouraged since this may cause the development of a 'sweet tooth' and influence the selection of cariogenic foods in later life. The use of a sucrose vehicle for vitamin supplements is also unwise, since these have been implicated in the aetiology of rampant caries in infants and young children. Above all, the child should never be given a dummy or bottle containing a sugar solution to be sucked at will, nor should a bottle of sweet drink be suspended in the cot so that the young child can drink at will throughout the night without waking the parent. This is likely to cause rampant caries (nursing-bottle caries) of the deciduous dentition (Figure 1.11, page 11).

5.11.6   Young children

Parents should be encouraged to give their children foods which do not foster a 'sweet tooth'. It is said that if children are given a savoury diet from an early age they will be happy to eat meals containing such foodstuffs in preference to sweet-tasting foods. Friends and relatives should be encouraged to bring small toys, fruit, or crisps as presents rather than sweets. Drinks at bedtime, other than water, should be strongly discouraged.

5.11.7   Chronically sick children

Many children with chronic medical disorders are placed at considerable risk when dental treatment procedures have to be carried out. Every care should be taken to prevent caries in such patients, although the syrupy vehicles often used to administer medicines make caries more likely. There is a need for strict dietary control as well as thorough oral hygiene, fluoride supplementation, and fissure sealing of susceptible teeth. Sugar-free medicines should be recommended.

5.11.8   Patients with dry mouths

This group is particularly at risk to dental caries, as discussed in Chapter 7. Thirst or the need to lubricate the mouth often results in the consumption of frequent sweet drinks or the chewing and sucking of sweets. Mouth lubricants and/or 'safe' drinks and sugar-free chewing gums should be recommended.

5.11.9   Dietary changes

Diet may remain constant over many years, but the dentist should watch for changes in caries status, and if a patient starts to develop new lesions the dietary cause should be sought. Perhaps the patient has left home, gone to boarding school, or started work and changed their diet radically. Alternatively, unemployment, retirement, bereavement, or illness may have resulted in changed dietary habits. Sometimes mints are substituted for cigarettes

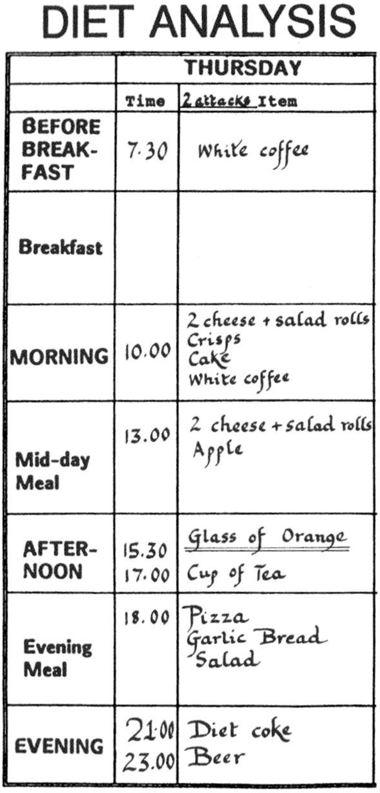

DIET ANALYSIS

	THURSDAY	
	Time	2 attacks Item
BEFORE BREAK-FAST	7.30	White coffee
Breakfast		
MORNING	10.00	2 cheese + salad rolls Crisps Cake White coffee
Mid-day Meal	13.00	2 cheese + salad rolls Apple
AFTER-NOON	15.30 17.00	Glass of Orange Cup of Tea
Evening Meal	18.00	Pizza Garlic Bread Salad
EVENING	21.00 23.00	Diet coke Beer

Figure 5.7. One day in the second diet sheet produced by the 24-year-old mechanical engineer. Figure 5.3 shows the original diet sheet and Figure 5.6 the suggestions for change agreed with the patient.

when someone gives up smoking, and the mint habit may persist long after the craving for a cigarette has gone. Mints sweetened with xylitol would be safe for teeth.

5.11.10   Monitoring the effect of dietary advice

Food intake and dietary habits are very difficult to influence. To find out whether the patient has followed the suggested dietary recommendations, the dentist can simply ask the patient about any changes. However, it is probably better to ask the patient to fill in another diet sheet. Figure 5.7 is a subsequent diet sheet filled in by the 'grazing' mechanical engineer (Figures 5.3 and 5.6) (see section 8.5.11). It would appear that this highly motivated young man had done all that had been suggested.

5.12   DIETARY MISCONCEPTIONS

A number of misconceptions exist about diet and dental caries, and it may be appropriate to end this chapter by laying a few ghosts! One serious misconception is that only refined carbohydrates (sucrose or white sugar) are harmful to teeth while other carbohydrates are not. Sucrose is certainly regarded as the 'arch-criminal' because it is the most abundant sugar. It is used by food manufacturers all over the world as a food ingredient and it is readily used by bacteria to form extracellular polysaccharides which make plaque thicker and stickier. However, other sugars, such as glucose, fructose, dextrose, glucose syrup, honey, corn syrup, invert sugar syrup, molasses, treacle, and maltose are also bad for teeth, although they may be somewhat less damaging than sucrose. In addition, brown sugar is just as bad as white.

Health foods are very fashionable nowadays; it has been suggested that fibrous foods such as apples and carrots 'clean' teeth, thus removing plaque and preventing caries. Although fibrous foods are preferable to a sucrose snack, there is no evidence that they can 'clean' the teeth. Another popular health food is honey. This so-called 'natural' sugar is just as cariogenic as other sugars. Many brands of muesli contain both sugar and honey. In the same way, the naturally occurring sugar in fruit juices makes these products just as cariogenic as fruit squashes.

Finally, it is very common for patients who are asked to give up sugar in tea and coffee to reduce the amount of sugar (say one teaspoon instead of two) rather than giving it up completely. Thus, the frequency of pH fall may not be altered. It is important to check that patients really understand the message, otherwise they may make a considerable effort to no avail (see section 8.3.1).

5.13 DOES DIETARY ADVICE WORK?

At the very end of the chapter it is slightly embarrassing to have to answer this direct and relevant question. Although the link between sugar and caries is irrefutable, there is no evidence that dietary advice at the individual level is effective.[11]

Does this then obviate the need for diet analysis and advice in general practice? Is it a waste of time? In the author's opinion it is not a waste of time, and to fail to consider diet, investigate it and advise the patient would be totally unethical. The patient may well reject the advice. That is their right. The teeth are theirs, not the dentist's. However, to leave a patient in ignorance of what a dentist considers is important to their dental health would be an abrogation of responsibility.

It is salutary for the dentist in the surgery to consider who else they may affect when they tell a particular patient about diet and dental caries. For instance, a mother may apply the information to her children, or a health worker in another discipline may also consider how the message is relevant to their work.

At the community level, dietary advice is very important, and since advice for dental health is in tune with that for general health, dentists should take every opportunity to deliver dental health messages. Thus campaigns to 'chuck sweets off the checkout', to remove fizzy drinks dispensers from school canteens, and opportunities to educate health visitors, nurses, and doctors about relevant dental health messages are invaluable. Such approaches potentially reach the whole population.

Further reading and references

1. Rugg-Gunn, A. J. (1993) *Nutrition and dental health*. Oxford University Press, Oxford.
2. Fejerskov, O. and Kidd, E. A. M. (eds) (2003) *Dental caries*. Ch.14: The role of dietary control. Blackwell Munksgaard, Oxford.
3. Rugg-Gunn, A. J., Hackett, A. F., Appleton, D. R., Jenkins, G. N., and Eastoe, J. E. (1984) Relationship between dietary habits and caries increment assessed over two years in 405 English adolescent school children. *Arch. Oral Biol.*, **29**, 983–992.
4. Burt, B. A., Eklund, S. A., Morgan, K. J., *et al.* (1988) The effects of sugar intake and the frequency of ingestion on dental caries increment in a three-year longitudinal study. *J. Dent. Res.*, **67**, 1422–1429.
5. Rugg-Gunn, A. J., Hackett, A. F., and Appleton, D. R. (1987) Relative cariogenicity of starch and sugars in a two-year longitudinal study of 405 English school children. *Caries Res.*, **21**, 464–473.
6. Downer, M. C. (1999) Caries experience and sucrose availability: an analysis of the relationship in the United Kingdom over fifty years. *Commun. Dent. Health*, **16**, 18–21.
7. Burt, B. and Pau, S. (2001) Sugar consumption and caries risk: a systematic review. *J. Dent. Educ.*, **65**, 1017–1023.
8. Moynihan, P. J. (2002) Dietary advice in dental practice. *Br. Dent. J.*, **193**, 563–568.
9. Gregory, J., Lowe, S., Bates, C. J., *et al.* (2000) National Diet and Nutrition Survey: young people aged 4–18 years. Volume 1: report of the diet and nutrition survey. HMSO, London.
10. Health Education Authority. (1996) *The scientific basis of dental health education*. A policy document, 4th edn. Health Education Authority, London.
11. Kay, E. J. and Locker, D. (1996) Is dental health education effective? A systematic review of current evidence. *Commun. Dent. Oral Epidemiol.*, **24**, 231–235.

6

Fluoride supplementation

6.1 INTRODUCTION

In 1901 an American dentist, Dr F. McKay, who had recently arrived in Colorado Springs from Pennsylvania, noticed that the teeth of many of his patients had a particular appearance which he called **mottled enamel**. He described this enamel as 'characterized by minute white flecks, or yellow or brown spots or areas, scattered irregularly or streaked over the surface of a tooth, or it may be a condition where the entire tooth surface is of a dead paper-white, like the colour of a china dish'.[1] It was not until the 1930s that research in the USA[2] and Britain[3] showed excessive fluoride in the drinking water (>2.0 parts per million (ppm F) or 2 mg F/litre) to be responsible for this mottling, and the condition was related to a low prevalence of dental caries. The term **dental fluorosis** was coined, and research was begun to study the possible benefits of fluoride.

In 1942 Dean and his co-workers[4] published the classical epidemiological studies carried out by the US Public Health Service on children aged 12–14 years living in 20 towns, relating caries experience and the fluoride content of the water supply. They showed that when the drinking water contained about 1 ppm of fluoride, the teeth of the lifelong inhabitants of that area had a low caries prevalence but no signs of dental fluorosis. For example, children aged 12–14 years had 50% less caries than those in areas with no fluoride in the water. These observations led to the addition of fluoride to fluoride-deficient water supplies in several controlled clinical studies throughout the world. The optimum level of fluoride recommended in temperate climates was 1 ppm while in tropical climates, where water consumption was greater, the level was reduced to 0.7 ppm. The results of these studies showed conclusively that it was possible to reduce caries by supplying optimal levels of fluoride. Since the early studies it has been clear that in order to continue to benefit from fluoridated water, it must continue throughout life. People moving into a fluoridated area after teeth have erupted also benefit.

However, many communities do not have piped water and for geographical and political reasons it has not been possible to fluoridate all water supplies. Consequently, a great deal of research has been carried out to develop alternative methods of supplementing fluoride intake. The aim of this chapter is to discuss this supplementation of fluoride in terms of efficacy and safety.

6.2 CRYSTALLINE STRUCTURE OF ENAMEL[5]

Enamel mineral is crystalline and has a lattice structure characteristic of hydroxyapatite, the smallest repeating unit of which can be expressed by the formula $Ca_{10}(PO_4)_6(OH)_2$. However, it is not a pure hydroxyapatite since it also has a non-apatite phase (amorphous calcium phosphate or carbonate) and additional ions or molecules are adsorbed onto the large surface area of the apatite crystals. It is important to understand that enamel is essentially a porous structure, allowing ions to diffuse into it. Indeed, the composition of its hydroxyapatite lattice can vary throughout, markedly affecting its structure. This can happen in several different ways:

- The crystal lattice has the capacity to substitute other ionic species of appropriate size and charge. Thus within the lattice, calcium can be exchanged for radium, strontium, lead, and hydrogen ions while phosphate can be exchanged for carbonate, and hydroxyl for fluoride.
- Sodium, magnesium, and carbonate can be substituted or absorbed at the crystal surface.
- There may be defects in the internal lattice.
- It is also possible for part of the lattice to be lost (demineralized) without the whole crystal disintegrating. Similarly, remineralization can occur.

6.2.1 Deposition of fluoride in enamel

There is a great deal of scope to affect the fluoride concentration of enamel since it can be deposited in three stages of enamel development. Low concentrations, reflecting the low levels of fluoride in tissue fluids, are incorporated in the apatite crystals during their formation. After calcification is complete, but before eruption, more fluoride is taken up by the surface enamel which is in contact with the tissue fluids. Finally, after eruption and throughout life, the enamel continues to take up fluoride from its external environment. At this time, the uptake of fluoride will be influenced by the state of the enamel, i.e. whether it is sound or whether acid-etching or caries have made it more porous by preferentially dissolving its interprismatic constituents. Any such increase in porosity facilitates the diffusion and uptake of fluoride by enamel. Enamel from newly erupted teeth also takes up more fluoride than mature enamel.

The fluoride content of intact surface enamel is much higher than the interior enamel but tends to be extremely variable. It varies between primary and permanent teeth, between different individuals living in the same area, between different teeth in the same individual, and even between different surfaces of the same tooth. In carious enamel, white-spot or brown-spot lesions, fluoride levels are raised, whereas in areas worn by attrition the levels are low.

6.3 DEMINERALIZATION AND REMINERALIZATION OF DENTAL HARD TISSUES

Caries is chemical dissolution of the dental hard tissues by the acid produced when bacteria degrade sugars. Under normal conditions the oral fluids are supersaturated with respect to both hydroxyapatite and fluorapatite. But, as pH is lowered in the plaque fluid below the critical pH of 5.5, plaque fluid becomes undersaturated with hydroxyapatite and a carious lesion forms. Because fluorapatite is less soluble than hydroxyapatite, plaque fluid remains supersaturated with respect to fluorapatite. This maintains the relative integrity of the surface layer (see Chapter 2, page 25).

Remineralization requires the presence of partially demineralized apatite crystals that can grow to their original size as a result of exposure to solutions supersaturated with respect to apatite. It is not common for entirely new crystals to form. Considerable remineralization of the surface of enamel in lesions free of plaque has been observed.

6.3.1 How does fluoride work in caries control?[5]

Fluoride works when it is present **in solution at the point of acid attack**. The fluoride interferes with the demineralization and remineralization processes. Fluoride reduces the rate of demineralization and enhances mineral uptake. It delays the progression of lesions and can thus be seen as an active chemical treatment for caries.

It is important to realize that fluoride incorporated into teeth during development does not necessarily result in an increased resistance of teeth to caries. Thus it is not correct to suggest that fluoride is only of benefit to children, or that it must be incorporated into developing enamel in order to have an effect. People of all ages benefit from fluoride because its action is topical, at the point of acid attack.

SOME IMPORTANT POINTS ABOUT FLUORIDE

- The predominant effect of fluoride is exerted topically
- For its effect to last, fluoride exposure must be continued
- Fluoride does not appear to have much influence on the initiation of a carious lesion, but can greatly retard its rate of progression
- Systemic absorption of fluoride during tooth development can result in dental fluorosis.

6.4 FLUOROSIS[6]

6.4.1 Signs of fluorosis

The first sign of excessive intake of fluoride during the period of tooth formation is the eruption of teeth with fluorosed or mottled enamel. Its appearance varies from fine white lines in the enamel to chalky, opaque enamel which turns brown or black after eruption. The enamel may even break apart soon after tooth eruption. Fortunately, this most severe form is unusual in the UK. The severity of change depends on the amount of fluoride ingested, its timing, and individual susceptibility due to factors such as body weight. The underlying histological feature is an increase in enamel porosity.

In order to see the early stages of fluorosis the teeth need to be cleaned and dried and examined in a good light. When fluorosis is mild, enamel merely

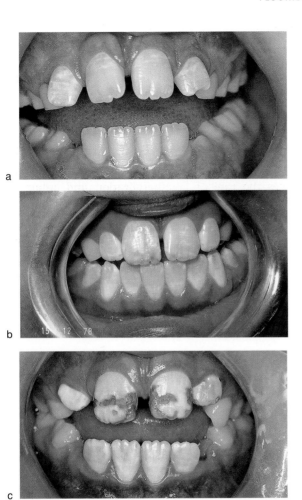

Figure 6.1. (a) Mild fluorosis. Note white flecks on upper anterior teeth.
(b) Moderate fluorosis. Note white striations and yellow-brown discolouration on
central incisors. (c) Severe fluorosis. Note loss of enamel.

loses its lustre and, when dried, opaque white flecks or patches can be seen
(Figure 6.1a). It is difficult to distinguish cases of mild fluorosis from other
opacities of enamel due to infections in childhood, genetic causes, or trauma.
However, such opacities are not usually aesthetically objectionable and it
has been suggested that the very early changes may actually enhance the
appearance of the teeth.

More obvious mottling or striations (Figure 6.1b), with or without yellow
or brown stains, are apparent in moderate cases of enamel fluorosis and are
not acceptable to patients or their parents. When the condition is very severe,
pitting occurs and the enamel is so hypoplastic that pieces break off very
easily (Figure 6.1c).

6.4.2 Mechanism of fluorosis[6]

Fluoride can induce dental fluorosis by affecting enamel maturation. The cumulated effect of ingested fluoride results in an impairment of mineral acquisition in the enamel during the long-lasting and complex process of enamel maturation.

Fluorosis can be caused by a single high dose of fluoride, by lower but multiple doses, and by low-level continuous exposure. Consequently it can be produced by ingestion of fluoride from the drinking-water (see Figure 6.2)[7] and toothpaste as well as by giving children fluoride tablets and drops.

Since the primary mode of action of fluoride is topical, little or no benefit is to be gained from swallowing it. Application methods should ensure elevated fluoride levels in the oral cavity. But the young should swallow as little fluoride as possible, so that the risk of fluorosis, particularly the cosmetically important forms, is minimized.

The risk of fluorosis depends on the fluoride dose relative to the weight of the child. For upper central incisors the risk is considered to be greatest for children between the ages of 15 and 30 months. When the first permanent molars erupt (at 6 years) the coronal development on the anterior teeth is nearly complete and ingestion of fluoride will have little impact on tooth development. Thus

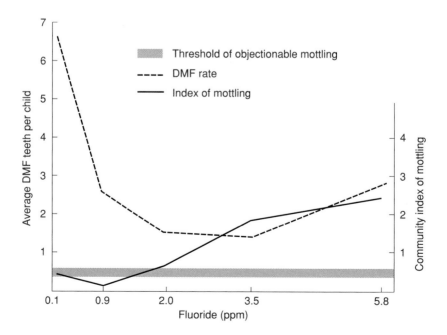

Figure 6.2. Fluoride content of water: caries experience and enamel mottling in British children aged 12–14 years. (From Forest (1956).[7] Reproduced courtesy of the Editor, *British Dental Journal.*

efforts to minimize fluoride ingestion need to be focused on children under the age of 7. As infants grow older and heavier, the risk of fluorosis moves to the more posterior teeth but because of the higher body weight, the dose of fluoride required to be ingested to cause fluorosis is greater.

It used to be considered that to be effective fluoride must be incorporated in developing enamel. For this reason it was suggested that children living in areas where there was minimal fluoride in the water should take fluoride systemically in the form of drops or tablets. Since it is now known that fluoride exerts its effect topically, this systemic use is no longer advocated. However, before this mechanism of action was understood, a number of children developed fluorosis by both taking fluoride tablets and using a fluoride toothpaste.

The fluorosis illustrated in Figure 6.1 was caused by excessive fluoride supplementation. The subjects all gave a history of supplemental fluoride drops or tablets at a daily dose of 0.5 mg F from birth to 2 years and 1 mg F thereafter, which was the dosage originally recommended before the advent of fluoridated toothpaste. Since these children were also having their teeth brushed with a fluoridated paste twice a day from the age of 6–8 months, it is not difficult to see why fluorosis resulted, as their total daily intake would have been in excess of 1.0 mg F.

The cases illustrated in Figure 6.1 suggest that there may be a variation in the response of these three children to fluoride. The histories revealed that there was also a variation in their ability to rinse and spit out after brushing. The child with severe fluorosis (Figure 6.1c) had difficulty rinsing until the age of 8 years. Therefore, in order to avoid fluorosis, it is necessary to restrict the quantity of fluoridated toothpaste used, particularly in children who live in an area where there is fluoride in the water. Figure 6.3 shows mild fluorosis in a child brought up in Birmingham, an area where the water is fluoridated.

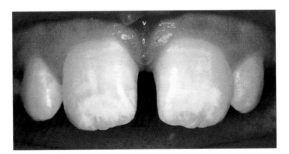

Figure 6.3. This patient shows mild fluorosis and spent his childhood in Birmingham, UK, where the water is artificially fluoridated. There is cloudy, diffuse mottling in the incisal third of the teeth, blending with the surrounding enamel. Cervically, horizontal white lines can be seen. (By courtesy of Dr Peter Rock).

6.5 WHICH FLUORIDE SUPPLEMENT?

Before considering supplementing fluoride, it is relevant to take into account the natural sources of fluoride in food. Seafood and tea are the principal dietary sources of this ion. In fish, it is the skin and bones which contain significant amount of fluoride. These parts of the fish become edible during canning, so canned fish may contain 9 ppm F. An average infusion of tea, depending on the brand, contains between 1.4 and 4.3 ppm F. Although consumption of tea in the UK is high, there is no evidence that this has a beneficial effect on the dental health of the population. This may be because sugar is frequently added to tea.

Fluoride in fish is relevant only if fish forms a major part of the diet. Similarly, only individuals consuming a very large volume of unsweetened tea might be expected to benefit dentally. Thus, for most people fluoride supplementation from foods is not practical and some other form of fluoride supplement should be considered.

To obtain the maximum benefit from fluoride, its transient presence is required soon after the initial caries attack. Since there is no way of knowing exactly when this occurs, the aim has to be regular and frequent exposure of the enamel to fluoride to arrest the early lesion. Indeed, there is clinical evidence to suggest that regular use of preparations containing low concentrations of fluoride is more effective than irregular use of agents containing higher concentrations. Furthermore, it has also been shown that when exposure to fluoride is discontinued, its caries-reducing effect gradually wanes. This is entirely logical, because fluoride is affecting the dynamics of lesion formation.

These factors have to be taken into consideration when choosing a fluoride supplement and the regime to be employed. Ultimately, however, the choice must be governed by the dental needs of the individual patient. Since available vehicles for fluoride supplementation contain varying amounts of fluoride, it is also necessary to consider the safety of the fluoride preparation chosen, in terms of fluorosis and toxicity.

Fluoride is used at home in toothpaste and mouthwashes, and/or applied in the dental surgery in the form of varnishes, topical solutions, and gels. If some of these preparations are accidentally swallowed during the period of tooth formation, there is a potential for fluorosis. Fluoride may also affect developing enamel if ingested as fluoridated water or fluoridated salt.

6.5.1 Fluoride in drinking water[6,8]

Fluoride occurs naturally in water supplies, usually at low concentrations (0.1–1.0 mg F/litre). Following the success of studies that artificially added fluoride to water supplies in the USA, schemes were implemented and evaluated in many parts of the world. Now, over 250 million people participate in water fluoridation programs in over 30 countries including USA, Canada, UK, Ireland, Brazil, Australia, and New Zealand. In the USA, more than 50% of the population receive fluoridated drinking water but in the UK only 10% of the population do, and many areas with high levels of dental caries (e.g. Northern Ireland, Scotland) remain excluded.

Studies evaluating the effect of water fluoridation on dental caries show a reduction in caries in both the deciduous and permanent dentitions of about 50%. However, most of these studies were undertaken before 1980. Since then it has become normal to use toothpaste containing fluoride, and this may explain why more recent comparisons between fluoridated and non-fluoridated communities show less dramatic results.

Water fluoridation is the most cost-effective public health measure to control dental caries. Provided piped domestic water systems serving large populations are available, it allows fluoride to be delivered cheaply to the majority of a community and the individuals benefit from the fluoride without any 'active' participation. Thus, it reaches those who are most difficult to access using other fluoride delivery methods.

However, this very accessibility of fluoride delivery has led to vigorous and sometimes passionate opposition to water fluoridation. The issue here is that once fluoride is added to the domestic water supply, consumers have little choice but to use it. This supposedly ethical argument may itself seem unethical, because in many parts of the world caries is worst in the most socially and economically deprived populations. Water fluoridation is one of the few interventions proven to reduce such oral health inequalities.

A number of studies have also considered the possible negative effects of water fluoridation, such as fluorosis. At the currently accepted optimal level, water fluoridation will result in some enamel mottling.

6.5.2 Salt fluoridation

The idea of adding fluoride to table salt originated in Switzerland, and fluoridated salt has been available in France, Germany, Costa Rica, Jamaica, Columbia and Hungary. The delivery system will potentially access the whole population but unlike water fluoridation, consumers have the choice of purchasing fluoridated or non-fluoridated salt. The weight of evidence suggests that salt fluoridation is probably effective, although it is difficult to design unbiased, randomized controlled clinical trials.

6.5.3 Fluoride in toothpaste[6,9]

Fluoride toothpaste is by far the most widely used method of applying fluoride. It is commonly used at home, but has also been used in community and school-based preventive programmes. A recent systematic review[10] concluded its use to be associated with a 24% reduction of caries in the permanent dentition of children and adolescents.[10] Only one study concerned deciduous teeth, showing a 37% reduction. The evidence to support the effectiveness of fluoride toothpaste is so compelling that it would now be considered unethical to use a non-fluoride toothpaste in a clinical trial.

It is important to remember that most of the above evidence has been gathered in clinical trials lasting 2–3 years. Thus the benefits accrued through a lifetime exposure may be substantially greater and mimic water fluoridation.

A number of factors are important in determining the effectiveness of fluoride toothpaste:
• frequency of use
• fluoride concentration
• rinsing behaviour
• time of day and duration of brushing.

Frequency of use

Those who claims to brush twice a day have lower caries levels than those who brush less frequently. Oral healthcare workers should advise brushing twice per day with a fluoride toothpaste.

Fluoride concentration

The effectiveness of fluoride toothpaste is concentration dependent. There is approximately a 6% reduction in caries for every increase of 500 ppm F and vice versa. Adult toothpastes generally contain 1000–1500 ppm F. However, a desire to reduce the potential risk of fluorosis has prompted the launch of children's toothpastes containing concentrations around 500 ppm F. These pastes provide less protection.

As a general rule, the author suggests that children under 6 should use an adult-concentration paste, but a small pea-sized portion of it. The child should be encouraged to spit out excess paste and not swallow it. Children's pastes (500 ppm F or less) could be recommended for children at low risk of caries living in an area where the water contains fluoride.

Today the fluoride agent in most toothpastes is either sodium fluoride or sodium monofluorophosphate. The abrasive used with sodium fluoride is silica, because a calcium abrasive would inactivate the fluoride. On the other hand, chalk-based abrasives can be used with sodium monofluorophosphate. Although the superiority of one fluoride agent over the other has been claimed, there is probably very little in it and both can be recommended. Table 6.1 gives the percentage by weight of sodium fluoride and sodium monofluorophosphate and the equivalent parts per million of fluoride. This is a useful table, because the labelling of the amount of fluoride in a paste may

Table 6.1. Percentage by weight of sodium fluoride and sodium monofluoro-phosphate toothpastes and equivalent parts per million fluoride[6]

Fluoride (ppm)	Sodium fluoride (% by weight)	Sodium monofluorphosphate (% by weight)
1500	0.32	1.14
1000	0.22	0.76
500	0.11	0.38

be given as % by weight rather than parts per million fluoride. This is confusing for the dentist trying to advise a patient, particularly as pastes formulated for children may have variable fluoride concentrations.

High-concentration fluoride pastes are also available (e.g. 2800 ppm F paste in the UK and 5000 ppm F paste in the USA). These products cannot be purchased over the counter but should be prescribed by a dentist on the practice notepaper or sold directly from the surgery. They are indicated for patients at high risk of caries, e.g. those presenting with multiple lesions, patients with root caries, or those with dry mouths. They should **never** be used in children because they will cause fluorosis and when they are prescribed for adults, patients should be warned not to allow children to use them.

Rinsing behaviour

There is some evidence that rinsing with large volumes of water after brushing reduces the effectiveness of fluoride toothpaste. Patients should therefore be advised to spit rather than rinse vigorously.

Time of day and duration of brushing

There is little evidence-based information on this. However, brushing last thing before bed potentially provides fluoride concentrations in saliva while the patient is asleep. Thus patients should brush before bed and at one other time during the day.

Fluorosis risk

The potential for fluorosis risk is from birth to 6 years with the aesthetically important upper incisors being at greatest risk between the ages of 15 and 30 months. The risk depends on the fluoride concentration of the toothpaste and the amount swallowed. The amount of paste on the brush (and thus potentially swallowed) is very important. Parents should place a small pea-sized smear of paste on the brush and encourage the child to spit out excess paste. Small children do not spit effectively, and the face of a 2-year-old is often level with the basin.

Toothpastes for patients with dry mouths

Patients with dry mouths find the taste of some pastes too astringent. Where possible, a paste without sodium lauryl sulphate and without a strong peppermint taste should be chosen. A high fluoride content may be advised for those developing carious lesions.

Toothpastes without fluoride

Although most toothpaste contains fluoride, it is astonishing to the author how many patients with multiple cavities are not using a fluoride toothpaste. Some do not brush their teeth. Others, because the cavities have made their teeth sensitive to hot and cold, select a toothpaste specifically formulated and advertised for sensitive teeth. In the UK the original flavour does not, at the time of writing, contain fluoride. Yet others, particularly those with a dry mouth, select a herbal toothpaste because it is not astringent. The paste is made with and without fluoride and sometimes, unluckily and unwittingly, the fluoride-free formulation is bought.

The moral of the story is that the dentist must check what toothpaste is being used, and when in doubt, ask to see it.

6.5.4 Fluoride mouthwashes

The daily or weekly use of a fluoride mouthwash is a valuable anticaries measure in high-risk patients who live in areas where the water supply is low in fluoride. The fluoride concentration advocated in the mouthwash depends on how frequently it is used. Individuals should rinse for 1 minute with 10 ml of a sodium fluoride solution at a concentration of 0.05% sodium fluoride if used once daily or at 0.2% if used at weekly intervals. A traditional literature review has suggested an average caries reduction of 30%.[11] Because of the lower fluoride concentration, daily rinsing is safer for children, provided that they are over 6 years old and can rinse adequately. For adults, choice should depend on patient cooperation. It is easy to forget to rinse weekly, but daily rinsing may become habitual.

Many fluoride rinses are available for sale over the counter in chemist shops and supermarkets. These products contain alcohol to stabilize the preparation, and peppermint to give a more astringent taste. The alcohol content can be as low as 4% (this would be equivalent to some beers) or as high as 27%. It is suggested that a bland tasting, alcohol-free mouthwash is chosen for children and patients with dry mouths who may find astringent mouthwashes intolerable. Where the alcohol content of the mouthwash is not stated on the bottle, the manufacturer should be contacted. There are some alcohol-free products on the market.

When combining mouthwashes with other fluoride therapies such as toothpaste, it is sensible to use the methods at different times of the day to obtain the greatest benefit.

USE OF MOUTHWASHES

Indications

The following patients should be encouraged to use mouthwashes:

- caries-prone children over the age of 6 years provided they can rinse and spit adequately
- patients with orthodontic appliances
- caries-prone adults, including those whose salivary flow rate has been reduced by drugs, disease, or radiotherapy
- adults with exposed root surfaces

Contraindications

- Mouthwashes should not be used by children under 6 years of age who are not capable of rinsing adequately.

The dietary history should always be obtained (see Section 5.10). Dietary advice, as well as oral hygiene instruction, should always precede a prescription for fluoride.

6.5.5 High-concentration preparations for periodic use

When dental apatite is exposed to preparations containing high concentrations of fluoride, the major reaction product is calcium fluoride (CaF_2). The slow dissolution and hence prolonged retention of CaF_2, particularly in the early carious lesion, is the key mechanism of the caries-reducing effect of concentrated topical fluoride.

Preparations come in various forms:

- sodium fluoride varnishes which are painted on in the surgery with a very small brush
- APF gels which are swabbed onto the tooth surface or applied in closely fitting trays.

The agents available, together with their respective fluoride concentrations and the amount of fluoride per ml, are listed in Table 6.2.

Table 6.2 Topical fluoride agents containing high concentrations of fluoride

Agents available	Concentration	mg F/ml
Sodium fluoride varnish	2.26% F	22
APF gel	1.23% F	12

USE OF FLUORIDE VARNISH

Indications

Twice yearly application of sodium fluoride varnish is indicated for the following groups of patients:

- Caries-prone adults who cannot or will not use a fluoride mouthwash
- Patients with removable orthodontic appliances and partial dentures (biannual applications)
- Children over 6 years and adults exposed to a greater cariogenic challenge because their dietary habits have changed since their last visit due to illness, change of school, or occupation
- Localized application to initial carious lesions where the clinician hopes to arrest progression of lesions and to protect vulnerable exposed root surfaces
- In exceptional cases, when it is difficult to control caries in children under 6 years, a small quantity of varnish may be carefully painted on each lesion followed by gentle washing with water

Contraindications

- Home use of fluoride varnish is contraindicated for safety reasons
- It is also generally contraindicated for children under the age of 6 years

Fluoride varnish

A recent systematic review[12] concluded that fluoride varnish reduced caries in the deciduous dentition by 33% and in the permanent dentition by 46% when compared with a placebo. It has also been shown to be effective in reducing root caries in high-risk adults. It is easy to apply safely, and requires minimal cooperation from the patient.

Duraphat, the product currently available in the UK, contains sodium fluoride in an alcoholic solution of natural varnishes. It is ideally applied on clean dry teeth with a brush, but it is water tolerant and will cling onto teeth even if moisture is present. Consequently, it is easier to apply than the other fluoride agents. The fluoride concentration is high (22 mg/ml), but the total amount of fluoride ingested is less than after gel application because only a small quantity needs to be applied. It has the added advantage that it need only be applied to vulnerable surfaces and not to the whole dentition.

Fluoride gels

Fluoride gels such as APF (acidulated phosphate fluoride) are now rarely used in the UK but they are still used in some countries and so are included here.

A systematic review suggested that fluoride gels, either professionally or self-applied, are associated with a 28% reduction in caries.[13] They have also been shown to decrease root caries in high-risk adults. The gels are usually applied by professionals but they can be self-applied under supervision. The gel is usually applied in a closely fitting tray for approximately 5 minutes, up to four times a year.

When the gel is applied in a tray, between 19 and 75% of the gel can be swallowed depending on whether a saliva ejector is used. If the gel is swallowed in sufficient quantity, it is very toxic (Table 6.3), so a very careful application technique must be employed. Its use is not generally recommended in the UK. However, if it is used the following guidelines should be observed.

- Trays should not be used for applying gels in children under 16 years of age; it is safer to swab the fluoride gel only on selected teeth.
- The dental chair should be upright and the patient should lean forward.
- The tray must be closely fitting and only a thin ribbon of gel, not more than 2 ml per tray, should be applied.
- A saliva ejector must be used.
- Patients should be instructed to spit out thoroughly immediately following application and suction should be used to evacuate the mouth.

6.6 TOXICITY

Anyone recommending the use of fluoride-containing dental preparations should be aware of the fluoride content and the potential hazards. Information on the toxicity of fluoride in humans is gathered from recorded cases of

Table **6.3** Toxicity of fluoride preparations, calculated for a 5-year-old child weighing 20 kg

	Sublethal acute poisoning dose	Potentially lethal poisoning dose
APF gel (1.23% F)	1.7 ml (1/3 teaspoon)	8 ml = 1.5 teaspoons
Sodium fluoride varnish (2.26% F)	0.9 ml (1/5 teaspoon)	4 ml = 4/5 teaspoon
Rinse		
0.2% NaF	22 ml (1/5 cup)	105 ml = 1 cup
0.05% NaF	88 ml (4/5 cup)	420 ml = 4 cups
Toothpaste[a]		
500 ppm	66 ml	200 ml
1000 ppm	33 ml	100 ml
1500 ppm	22 ml	66 ml

[a] *Tubes of toothpaste generally contain 50, 100, or 125 ml.*

deliberate or accidental overdosage. The acute lethal dose is approximately 15 mg/kg body weight, although as little as 5 mg/kg may kill some children. A dose of 5 mg/kg should trigger immediate emergency treatment. As little as 1 mg/kg can produce sublethal toxic effects.

The exact mechanism by which fluoride produces its toxic effect is not known. Symptoms of sublethal poisoning are salivation, nausea, and vomiting. The symptoms usually appear within an hour of ingestion and, if overdosage occurs as a result of topical fluoride application, may not be manifest until the patient has left the surgery. Death from respiratory or cardiac failure occurs within 24 hours of a lethal dose.

A small quantity of fluoride (less than 5 mg/kg body weight) is neutralized by drinking a large volume of milk. However, if more than 5 mg/kg has been ingested or if there is any doubt about the exact quantity consumed, the child should be taken to hospital and given gastric lavage. Speed is of the utmost importance because fluoride is very rapidly absorbed.

Table 6.3 lists some of the fluoride agents in use, the amount required to produce early toxic effects and the potential lethal dose—all in relation to the average 5-year-old weighing about 20 kg (44 lb). These values would be considerably lower for the average 2-year-old. For a 5-year-old, as little as one third of a teaspoonful of APF gel can produce toxic effects and $1^{1}/_{2}$ teaspoonfuls can be lethal. Sodium fluoride varnish is even more concentrated; less than a teaspoonful is dangerous for a young child.

Consequently, if fluoride varnish is used in exceptional cases in preschool children, extreme care must be exercised. For children over the age of 6 years, a fluoride varnish should be chosen because, although the fluoride concentration is high, only a small quantity is applied and, unlike gels in trays, a safe technique requires minimal cooperation from a child.

Although no cases of acute toxicity due to ingestion of toothpaste have ever been reported, a 5-year-old could be severely poisoned by consuming about two thirds of a 100 ml tube of 1500 ppm fluoride paste; a 1-year-old would need to consume only half this amount. Fluoride toothpaste should therefore be kept out of the reach of young children, and this is particularly important with the advent of the new high-fluoride pastes for use by adults at high risk of caries. Similarly, fluoride mouthwashes should be kept out of reach of younger children.

Further reading and references

1. McKay, F. S. (1916) An investigation into mottled teeth. (1). *Dent. Cosmos.*, **58**, 477–484.

2. Churchill, H. V. (1931) The occurrence of fluorides in some waters of the United States. *J. Dent. Res.*, **12**, 141–148.
3. Ainsworth, N. J. (1933) Mottled teeth. *Br. Dent. J.*, **55**, 233–250.
4. Dean, H. T., Arnold, F. A., and Evolve, E. (1942) Domestic water and dental caries, V. Additional studies of the relation of fluoride domestic waters to dental caries experience in 4, 425 white children aged 12–14 years, of 13 cities in 4 States. *Public Health Rep.*, **57**, 1155–1179.
5. Fejerskov, O. and Kidd, E. A. M. (eds) (2003) *Dental caries*. Ch.4: Clinical interactions between the tooth and oral fluids. Blackwell Munksgaard, Oxford.
6. Fejerskov, O. and Kidd, E. A. M. (eds) (2003) *Dental caries*. Ch.13: Clinical use of fluoride. Blackwell Munksgaard, Oxford.
7. Forest, J. R. (1956) Caries experience and enamel defects in areas with different levels of fluoride in the drinking water. *Br. Dent. J.*, **100**, 195–200.
8. McDonagh, M., Whiting, P. F., Wilson, P. M. *et al.* (2000) Systematic review of water fluoridation. *BMJ*, **321**, 855–859. (See also http//www.york.ac.uk/inst/crd/fluorid.htm).
9. Davies, R. M. (2003) The prevention of dental caries and periodontal disease from the cradle to the grave: what is the best available evidence? *Dent. Update*, **30**, 170–179.
10. Marinho, V. C., Sheiham, A., Logan, S., and Higgins, J. P. (2003) Fluoride toothpastes for preventing dental caries in children and adolescents. (Cochrane Review). In: *The Cochrane Library, Issue 1*. Update Software, Oxford (see also: http://www.cochrane.org).
11. Ripa, L. W. (1991) A critique of topical fluoride methods (dentifrices, mouthrinses, operator-, and self-applied gels) in an era of decreased caries and increased fluorosis prevalence. *J. Publ. Health Dent.*, **51**, 23–41.
12. Marinho, V. C. C. *et al.* (2002) Fluoride varnishes for preventing dental caries in children and adolescents (Cochrane Review). In: *The Cochrane Library, Issue 3*. Update Software, Oxford (see also:http://www.cochrane.org).
13. Marinho, V. C. C. *et al.* (2003) Fluoride gels for preventing dental caries in children and adolescents (Cochrane Review). In: *The Cochrane Library, Issue 1*. Update Software, Oxford (see also:http://www.cochrane.org).

Saliva and caries

7.1 INTRODUCTION

Saliva is a complex oral fluid consisting of a mixture of secretions from the major salivary glands and the minor glands of the oral mucosa. Ninety per cent of saliva is produced by the three pairs of major glands: parotid, submandibular, and sublingual. The rest of it is produced by thousands of minor salivary glands distributed throughout the mouth and throat. Most of the saliva is produced at meal times as a response to stimulation due to tasting and chewing (stimulated saliva). For the rest of the day, although salivary flow is low, it is extremely important. In healthy individuals under resting conditions, without the stimulation associated with chewing, there is a constant slow flow of saliva which moistens and helps to protect the teeth, tongue, and mucous membranes of the mouth and oropharynx (resting saliva). The flow rate peaks during the afternoon and virtually stops during sleep. This has important clinical implications for the timing of oral hygiene. Since plaque and food debris and a greatly reduced salivary flow provide ideal conditions for dental caries, the most important time of day to clean teeth is at night before going to sleep.

The normal resting or unstimulated secretion rate in adults is between 0.3 and 0.5 ml per minute. The normal stimulated secretion rate in adults is 1–2 ml per minute. However, the rates may be reduced to less than 0.1 ml per minute or may not be measurable in individuals with severe salivary gland malfunction. In less severe cases of hyposalivation the stimulated secretion rate is between 0.7 and 1.0 ml per minute. The term **xerostomia** is used to describe the perception of a dry mouth, but 50% of salivary function must be lost before the subjective changes are recognized. Thus a patient may be unaware of reduced salivary flow. The clinical implication is that it is important to measure salivary flow, because it may be low and the patient may be unaware of this.

The composition and viscosity of saliva depends on the relative contributions from the various salivary glands. Although they are similar in structure, the viscosity of the secretions they produce varies. Parotid secretions are watery and clear, whereas the minor glands in the mouth and throat produce secretions that are more viscous and ropy. The secretions produced by the submandibular and sublingual glands are respectively two and three times more viscous than parotid saliva. Under normal conditions the parotid glands produce 50% of the stimulated saliva and 20% of the resting saliva. Most of the resting saliva is produced by the submandibular (65%), sublingual (7–8%) and minor salivary glands (7–8%). Resting saliva is therefore more viscous than stimulated saliva. It becomes even more viscous and ropy when only the minor glands contribute. Such saliva is uncomfortable for the patient, because it makes swallowing difficult.

7.2 SALIVA AND DENTAL HEALTH[1]

7.2.1 Functions of saliva

Although saliva aids swallowing and digestion, and is required for optimal function of the taste buds, its most important role is to maintain the integrity of the teeth, tongue, and mucous membranes of the oral and oropharyngeal regions. Its protective action is manifested in several ways:

- It forms a protective mucoid coating on the mucous membrane which acts as a barrier to irritants and prevents desiccation.
- Its flow helps to clear the mouth of food and cellular and bacterial debris and consequently retards plaque formation.
- It is capable of regulating the pH of the oral cavity by virtue of its bi-carbonate content as well as its phosphate and amphoteric protein con-stituents. An increase in secretion rate usually results in an increase in pH and buffering capacity. The mucous membrane is thus protected from acid in food or vomit. In addition the fall in plaque pH, as a result of the action of acidogenic organisms, is minimized.
- It helps to maintain the integrity of teeth in several ways because of its calcium and phosphate content. It provides minerals which are taken up by the incompletely formed enamel surface soon after eruption (post-eruptive maturation). Tooth dissolution is prevented or retarded and remineralization is enhanced by the presence of a copious salivary flow. The film of glyco-protein formed on the tooth surface by saliva (the acquired pellicle) may also protect the tooth by reducing wear due to erosion and abrasion.
- Saliva is capable of considerable antibacterial and antiviral activity by virtue of its content of specific antibodies (secretory IgA) as well as lysozyme, lactoferrin, and lactoperoxidase.

7.2.2 Causes of reduced salivary flow

There are numerous systemic conditions (listed in the box overleaf) which can alter the salivary flow rate. However, the most serious causes of mal-function of the salivary glands are radiotherapy in the region of these glands, drugs, and disease.

Radiotherapy

The exposure of the salivary glands to radiation during radiotherapy for neo-plasms in the head and neck region usually results in a severe reduction in salivary flow (less than 0.1 ml/min.). When the parotid glands are involved, there is also a considerable increase in its total protein content resulting in a thick, viscous secretion which makes the condition even more uncomfort-able. The time taken for salivary flow rate to return towards normal values varies and depends on the individual as well as the dose to which the glands have been exposed. Thus, in some patients, there is a considerable improve-ment after 3 months while in others hyposalivation may be permanent as a result of atrophy of the glands induced by the radiation.

Drugs

A large number of therapeutic drugs affect salivary flow rate as well as its composition. The groups of drugs which result in decreased flow are listed in

SYSTEMIC CAUSES OF 'DRY MOUTH'

- Drugs
- Psychological factors
- Sjögren's syndrome
- Hormonal changes (pregnancy, post-menopause)
- Diabetes mellitus
- Dehydration
- Neurological diseases
- Pancreatic disturbances
- Liver disturbances
- Nutritional deficiencies (anorexia nervosa, malnutrition)
- Systemic lupus erythematosus
- Immunodeficiency disease (AIDS)
- Duct calculi
- Smoking
- ?Ageing

the box opposite. Consequently, if any of them are used for more than a few weeks, steps must be taken to protect the teeth from caries. In addition, chemotherapy with cytotoxic drugs used in the management of some malignancies may also cause acute onset of dry mouth.

Disease

Acute and chronic inflammation of the salivary glands (sialadenitis), benign or malignant tumours, as well as Sjögren's syndrome, may all lead to hyposalivation depriving the individual of the protective action of saliva. Sjögren's syndrome is an autoimmune connective tissue disorder. It affects principally the salivary and lacrymal glands which become damaged by lymphocytic infiltrates and therefore produce less secretion. Fifteen to thirty per cent of patients with rheumatoid arthritis also have Sjögren's syndrome. For this reason the possibility of a dry mouth should be considered in patients with rheumatoid arthritis.

Age

It is generally assumed that a reduction in salivary flow is the inevitable result of ageing. However, recent studies show that, at least for the parotid gland flow, there is no diminution of stimulated fluid output with increasing age in healthy subjects not on therapeutic drugs. On the other hand, there is some evidence that atrophic changes can occur in submandibular and minor

MEDICATIONS THAT RETARD SALIVARY FLOW

- Anticholinergics
- Antidepressants
- Antiemetics
- Antihistamines
- Antihypertensives
- Antinauseants
- Antiparkinsonian drugs
- Antipsychotic drugs
- Appetite suppressants
- Diuretics
- Expectorants
- Hypnotics
- Muscle relaxants
- Tranquilizers

glands with age, which could result in a feeling of dryness even when the flow rate of stimulated saliva is normal. It would seem, therefore, that any small decrease in salivary flow as a result of ageing is very slight compared with reductions in flow due to disease and the use of drugs in this group of individuals.

7.2.3 General consequences of reduced salivary flow

The useful role of saliva is not usually appreciated until there is a shortage. The contribution that saliva makes to oral health is therefore best demonstrated by examining the consequences of hyposalivation. The oral mucosa, without the lubricating and protective action of saliva, is more prone to traumatic ulceration and infection. Mucositis presents as tenderness, pain, or a burning sensation and is exacerbated by spicy foods, fruits, alcoholic and carbonated beverages, hot drinks, and tobacco. Taste sensation is altered, and chewing and swallowing present difficulties, particularly if the food is bulky or dry. When salivary flow is diminished, foods requiring a great deal of chewing are not well tolerated. This makes matters worse because chewing itself helps to stimulate salivary flow, provided there is some glandular activity left. Speaking may become difficult because of lack of lubrication. These individuals also suffer from extreme sensitivity of teeth to heat and cold, especially if any dentine is exposed. Edentulous patients may have problems tolerating dentures, probably because of reduction in surface tension between the dry mucosa and the fitting surface of the denture.

There is an increase in dental plaque accumulation, which makes gingivitis more likely. However, there is no evidence that periodontitis, which involves loss of bone support, is affected. There is also modification of the plaque flora in favour of *Candida*, mutans streptococci, and lactobaccilli. Consequently, in patients with dry mouths, candidal infections are frequent and rampant caries is common if no preventive measures are taken. Radiation caries is discussed in detail later (see section 7.4.2).

7.3 CLINICAL MANAGEMENT OF 'DRY MOUTH'

7.3.1 Assessment

Drug history

As a first step, the patient's drug history should be checked since all the medications listed in the box on page 131 can adversely affect salivary flow and consequently aggravate the problem. New formulations are often prescribed so it is always wise to check with the British National Formulary for any side effects. If any of these drugs are being taken for long periods it may be advisable for a dentist to contact the patient's medical practitioner to see whether the drug regime could be modified.

It is also relevant to check whether the patient is using a mouthwash, since some of them contain up to 27% alcohol and mint flavourings that can cause further discomfort. If the alcohol content of a mouthwash is not stated on the bottle, the dentist should contact the manufacturer for this information.

Salivary flow measurements

It is important to standardize the time of day at which saliva is collected, since the flow rate peaks during the afternoon. The patient should not eat or drink (except water) for at least 1 hour before collection. Measurement of unstimulated and stimulated flow rates should be determined as described in section 3.7.5. This will help to assess the extent of the problem by providing a quantitative assessment of an individual's salivary gland function and can be used to monitor the course of the disease. A simple comparison of the stimulated and unstimulated rate will indicate if the glands are capable of being stimulated.

7.3.2 Conservative measures to relieve symptoms

Relief from oral dryness and its accompanying discomfort can be achieved conservatively by:
- sipping water frequently all day long
- restricting intake of substance that exacerbate dryness such as cigarettes, caffeine-containing drinks, and alcohol
- avoiding astringent products such as alcohol-containing or strong mint-flavoured mouthwashes, strongly flavoured toothpastes

- coating the lips with lip salve or Vaseline
- humidifying the sleeping area.

7.3.3 Salivary stimulants

Having established the extent of impairment, the next step is to try to increase salivary flow.

Salivary stimulants will only be helpful when there is some glandular activity present. The following agents have been used:

- Chewing a sugar-free gum, particularly one containing xylitol and or chlorhexidine, will increase salivary flow safely (see page 103). Sucking acidic sweets may also increase salivary flow. However, if a patient is dentate anything sugar-containing or acidic is contraindicated. Some fruit drops flavoured with artificial sweeteners, normally marketed for diabetics, will not cause caries but are very acidic and may dissolve enamel and dentine.
- SST (Sinclair) is a saliva-stimulating tablet which is sucked. It increases secretion of saliva through physiological stimulation of the taste buds. The tablet contains sorbitol, citric acid, citric acid salts, and a phosphate buffer. It is formulated with the buffer so that it does not damage teeth.
- Salivix (Provalis) is a proprietary lozenge containing malic acid, gum arabic, calcium lactate, sodium phosphate, lycasin, and sorbitol. The manufacturers claim that it stimulates salivary flow and that, because of the calcium lactate buffer present, it does not demineralize enamel in spite of a pH of 4.0.

The systemic use of drugs such as pilocarpine hydrochloride has proved successful in stimulating saliva.[3] However, it does not restore lost glandular function and should be used with caution because of potential unpleasant side effects. Pilocarpine reproduces the effects of widespread stimulation of the parasympathetic nervous system. Consequently, as well as stimulating saliva and tear production, it can cause sweating, flushing, nausea, and diarrhoea. It can also slow the pulse rate, producing a fall in blood pressure and cause reflex narrowing of airways. It is therefore contraindicated in patients with cardiac or chest problems. The recommended dose is one 5 mg tablet daily. Once the patient has learnt to tolerate the side effects, the dose may be increased up to three 5 mg tablets daily, which is the therapeutic dose. The maximum effect is not noted until at least 30 minutes after swallowing the tablet. The effect lasts for 60–120 minutes.

7.3.4 Saliva substitutes

In the past, individuals with a dry mouth have had to rely on frequent moistening with water. Several saliva substitutes are now available to make the patient feel more comfortable and ideally to supply calcium, phosphate, and fluoride ions to aid remineralization. Saliva substitutes have been produced in the form of sprays, lozenges, or mouthwashes.

Sprays to give viscosity

The following preparations are commercially available in the UK: Luborant (Antigen International Ltd), Saliva Orthana (A S Pharma), Glandosane (Fresenius Kabi) and Saliveze (Wyvern). They all contain calcium, phosphate, sodium, magnesium, and potassium ions. However, while Luborant, Glandosane and Saliveze contain carboxymethylcellulose to provide viscosity, Saliva Orthana contains mucin prepared from the gastric mucosa of the pig. The other important difference between them is that while Luborant and Saliva Orthana both contain fluoride, have a pH between 6 and 7 and have been shown to have a significant remineralizing capacity *in vitro*, Saliveze and Glandosane do not contain fluoride. Glandosane has a somewhat lower pH at 5.1 and should, therefore, be used only for edentulous patients. The sprays should be directed towards the inside of the cheeks and not down the throat. A clinical trial comparing a mucin-based saliva substitute to a mucin-free placebo in patients with advanced malignant disease with dry mouth, found no difference between the two saliva substitutes.[3]

Lozenges

Lozenges are only helpful if there is enough saliva present to dissolve them. Saliva Orthana is also available in the form of a lozenge. It does not contain fluoride but is quite palatable.

Products containing antimicrobial proteins

Dentifrices, mouthrinses, and gels are on the market in several countries containing antimicrobial proteins such as peroxidose, lysozyme, and lactoferrins. The objective is to compensate for the lack of host- mediated protection derived from these proteins in those with normal salivary flow. Examples are the Biotene (Anglian) and bioXtra (Molar) product ranges.

Viscous or ropy saliva

When saliva is present but is ropy, rinsing or gargling with a mouthwash made up by mixing half a teaspoonful of baking powder with one litre of warm water will break up the mucous in the mouth and throat. This can help patients with mild mucositis due to radiotherapy.

Unfortunately, there has been no controlled study to date comparing the acceptability and effectiveness of these preparations, so no particular one can be recommended. Indeed, none of these agents is ideal and some patients still resort to filling a spray bottle with water to be used at frequent intervals. However, it is obvious that any preparation with an unbuffered, low pH should never be used for dentate patients. Ideally, the saliva substitute should contain fluoride and be supplemented by a daily fluoride mouthwash (see page 120).

7.4 SALIVA AND CARIES

7.4.1 Anticariogenic actions of saliva

Theoretically saliva can influence the carious process in several ways (see box).

Although there is no doubt that saliva possesses all the anticaries properties listed below, research workers have been frustrated in their attempts to directly relate any particular salivary factor to the incidence of caries. One of the reasons for their failure is the fact that caries is a process occurring intermittently, in which host, microorganisms, and substrate are all involved. Since saliva has the ability to affect all of them in several different ways, it becomes easy to understand the difficulties encountered in trying to evaluate any single anticaries factor at any one time. Nevertheless, there is sufficient evidence to demonstrate a negative correlation between buffering capacity of stimulated and unstimulated whole saliva and caries. In addition, there is no doubt that when saliva is absent, or drastically reduced in

---

HOW SALIVA INFLUENCES THE CARIOUS PROCESS

- The flow of saliva can reduce plaque accumulation on the tooth surface and also increase the rate of carbohydrate clearance from the oral cavity.

- The diffusion into plaque of salivary components such as calcium, phosphate, hydroxyl, and fluoride ions can reduce the solubility of enamel and promote remineralization of early carious lesions.

- The carbonic acid–bicarbonate buffering system, as well as ammonia and urea constituents of the saliva, can buffer and neutralize the pH fall which occurs when plaque bacteria metabolize sugar. The pH and buffering capacity of saliva is related to its secretion rate. The pH of parotid saliva increases from about 5.5 for unstimulated saliva to about 7.4 when the flow rate is high. The respective pH values for submandibular saliva are 6.4 and 7.1. An increase in the secretion rate of saliva also results in a greater buffering capacity. In both cases this is due to the increase in sodium and bicarbonate concentrations.

- Several non-immunological components of saliva such as lysozyme, lactoperoxidase, and lactoferrin have a direct antibacterial action on plaque microflora or may affect their metabolism so that they become less acidogenic.

- Immunoglobulin A (IgA) molecules are secreted by plasma cells within the salivary glands, while another protein component is produced in the epithelial cells lining the ducts. The total concentration of IgA in saliva may be inversely related to caries experience.

- Salivary proteins could increase the thickness of the acquired pellicle and so help to retard the movement of calcium and phosphate ions out of enamel.

quantity, caries can be rampant. Hence caries preventive measures must be taken when there is any interference in salivary function which diminishes flow and when buffering capacity is low.

7.4.2 Radiation caries[4]

Following radiotherapy for tumours in the vicinity of the salivary glands, or chemotherapy with cytotoxic drugs, conditions conducive to a rapid onset of caries are created not only by the shortage of saliva but also by the resultant dietary change. Liquids and soft foods, high in carbohydrate content, are often consumed at frequent intervals throughout the day. To make matters worse there is also an alteration in the oral flora in favour of cariogenic organisms such as mutans steptococci and lactobaccilli as well as *Candida*[5] which can exacerbate the mucositis caused by the irradiation. If no special preventive regime is followed, rampant caries is very likely to develop.

It is now know that X-radiation in the doses administered in cancer therapy does not physically alter enamel to increase its caries susceptibility. Indeed, laboratory studies have demonstrated that irradiated enamel is more resistant than non-irradiated enamel to an artificial caries attack or de-mineralization. It has also been shown *in vivo* that teeth are severely affected only if the main salivary glands are within the radiation field so that there is a drastic reduction in saliva flow.

The typical pattern of caries development is shown in Figures 1.10 and 7.1. The incisal edges of anterior teeth and the cusp tips of posterior teeth,

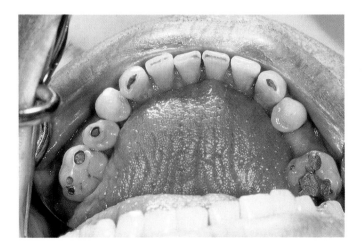

Figure 7.1. A typical pattern of carious attack in a patient with xerostomia, in this case caused by radiotherapy in the region of the salivary glands. The cusp tips and incisal edges are typically attacked because dentine is often exposed by tooth wear in these area. Dentine is more susceptible to caries than enamel.

which are normally very resistant to carious attack, suffer rapid destruction. The cervical margins of the teeth are also highly susceptible. All these areas are covered by only a thin layer of enamel, or the enamel may have been worn away so that, without the protection of saliva, caries rapidly invades dentine. If any root surfaces are exposed they are even more rapidly attacked and are very difficult to restore. It is very important that caries is controlled, because extractions can result in osteoradionecrosis or 'bone death' caused by radiation. This is due to a reduction in the osteocyte population and in the vascularity of the bone. Such changes make the bone vulnerable to trauma and infection, and impair its capacity to remodel and repair after extractions.

7.4.3 Management of dentate patients following radiotherapy for head and neck cancers

A regime to control caries and periodontal disease is vital in order to avoid the need for extractions. Salivary flow is diminished, particularly during the first year, increasing the risk of caries and the periodontium has lowered biological potential for healing.

For periodontal disease

It is essential to maintain healthy periodontal tissues since they offer a route for infection to the bone. Patients should therefore be monitored closely every 3–4 months when oral hygiene instruction is reinforced and scaling carried out when necessary. This emphasis on oral hygiene will also aid caries control.

For caries

Several studies show that, without dietary restrictions, caries can be successfully controlled by daily 5-minute self-applications of a 1% sodium fluoride gel in custom-made applicator trays. However, this level of commitment is difficult to achieve. When patients do not comply fully with such a regime, caries is uncontrolled, particularly where both parotids have been irradiated. Fortunately a simpler regime is now possible because of the availability of the antibacterial agent chlorhexidine which is an effective plaque inhibitor and anticaries agent. Studies combining the use of fluoride and chlorhexidine have been successful in caries control after radiotherapy.[6,7] Based on the results of these studies, some simple strategies are recommended (see box).

7.4.4 Preventive measures for patients with dry mouths

The same fundamental steps that have to be taken before putting into practice any preventive measures also apply to these patients. The dentist must first recognize that a patient is 'at risk' (see section 3.8); the situation must be

CARIES CONTROL STRATEGIES

- The patient should see the dentist at least every 3 months. Plaque control needs to be excellent, and professional plaque control should be considered (see page 80).

- Until salivary flow returns to normal limits, the risk of caries is high. Therefore, stimulated flow rates should be measured every 3–4 months to help to establish the level of caries risk (see section 3.7.5).

- Rigid dietary control is impractical. However, each time the patient is seen, the opportunity should be taken to reinforce the importance of avoiding sweet drinks and snacks. The bedtime sweet drink is particularly dangerous. Taste sensation is lost during radiotherapy but when it returns, 2–4 months later, there often is a sudden craving for sweet foods and drinks. Patients should also be discouraged from attempts to stimulate salivary flow by sucking sweets. Instead, chewing a sugar-free gum containing xylitol will be safer and more effective. The use of a saliva substitute until salivary flow returns will also be helpful.

- Patients should use a sodium fluoride (0.05% NaF) mouthrinse daily for several years to help arrest any initial carious lesions. It will also help to alleviate sensitivity from pre-existing areas of exposed dentine which have lost the protective action of saliva. A low-alcohol or water-based product with a mild taste should be chosen (see section 6.5.4).

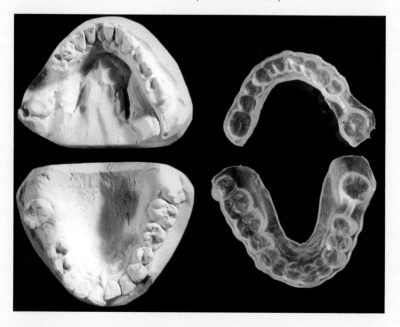

Figure 7.2. Custom-made flexible, vacuum-moulded trays for self-application of chlorhexidine or fluoride gel.

CARIES CONTROL STRATEGIES—cont'd.

- A 1% chlorhexidine gel (Corsodyl) should be applied by the patient in custom-made applicator trays (Figure 7.2) for 5 minutes every night for 14 days. This is repeated every 3–4 months until salivary flow returns to normal. Such treatment has been shown to keep the level of mutans streptococci in control for at least 3 months.[7] Compliance with this regime can be checked before and after treatments by use of proprietary kits to measure levels of mutans streptococci. Any possible chlorhexidine staining can be removed when these patients are seen at their regular recall visits. It is important to note that chlorhexidine is inactivated by sodium lauryl sulphate, the detergent present in most toothpastes. Patients should therefore be instructed to rinse toothpaste out thoroughly before any application of chlorhexidine.
- Any patient with a dry mouth should avoid smoking, alcohol, and caffeine-based drinks since any of these can exacerbate the problem.

explained to the patient and the patient must then be encouraged to adopt the following necessary preventive measures.

Plaque caontrol

Excellent plaque control is very important. It should be explained to the patient that the risk of caries is high and their cleaning should be of 'gold medal standard' because anything less is unlikely to be good enough to prevent caries. The support of a hygienist and professional plaque control can be invaluable.

Dietary control

To alleviate the dryness in their mouths, these patients are tempted to suck sweets or drink sweet drinks at frequent intervals. It is therefore particularly important that after a diet analysis (see section 5.10), the patient should be given dietary advice (see section 5.11). Particular attention should be given to the restriction of refined carbohydrate to meal times and avoiding a sweet drink at bedtime. The use of sugar-free chewing gum should be encouraged.

The use of fluoride

A daily sodium fluoride (0.05% NaF) mouthwash should be recommended in the long term, together with topical application of a fluoride varnish on any vulnerable sites by the dentist every 6 months.

Chlorhexidine gel application

When the shortage of saliva is not severe, good plaque control with a fluoride-containing toothpaste, dietary control and the use of fluoride may be the only measures required. In extreme cases chlorhexidine gel application every 3–4 months, as outlined for radiotherapy patients, is also necessary.

Without constant vigilance and regular monitoring by the dentist, a short lapse by the patient may have disastrous results.

Further reading and references

1. Kidd, E. A. M. and Fejerskov, O. (eds) (2003) *Dental caries*. Ch. 2: Secretion and composition of saliva. Blackwell Munksgaard, Oxford.
2. Edgar, W. M. and O'Mullane, D. M.(1990) *Saliva and dental health*. British Dental Journal, London.
3. Brennen, M. T., Shariff, G., Lockhart, P. B., and Fox, P. C. (2002) Treatment of xerostomia: a systematic review of therapeutic trials. *Dent. Clin. N. Am.*, **46**, 847–856.
4. Joyston-Bechal, S. (1992) Management of oral complications following radiotherapy. *Dent. Update*, **19**, 232–238.
5. Brown, L. R., Dreizen, S., Handler, S., and Johnston, D. A. (1975) Effect of radiation-induced xerostomia on human oral microflora. *J. Dent. Res.*, **54**, 740–750.
6. Katz, S. (1982) The use of fluoride and chlorhexidine for the prevention of radiation caries. *J. Am. Dent. Assoc.*, **104**, 164–170.
7. Joyston-Bechal, S., Hayes, K., Davenport, E., and Hardie, J. M. (1992). Caries, mutans streptococci and lactobacilli in irradiated patients during a 12 month programme using chlorhexidine and fluoride. *Caries Res.*, **26**, 384–90.

Patient communication and motivation

8.1 THE ESSENTIAL ROLE OF THE PATIENT

The last three chapters have discussed the management of dental caries by the removal of plaque by the patient, control of diet, and the use of fluoride supplements at home. The success of all these strategies depends on the patient, but it is a well-known fact that patients frequently choose not to comply with health advice given to them. Many know they should lose weight, take more exercise, finish their course of antibiotics, practice 'safe' sex, give up smoking, but choose not to.

A number of factors are known to influence compliance (see box). Thus oral health behaviours should not be assessed in isolation from considerations of the patient's overall lifestyle, circumstances, beliefs, knowledge, and attitudes. A lot of time and effort is spent on giving advice to patients, and this is costly. If the advice is seemingly ignored by the patient it can lead to frustration and increasing dissatisfaction for members of the dental team, quite apart from the fact that the patient's disease level remains unaltered.

Throughout the text it has been stated that the carious process can be modified by altering diet, use of fluoride, and improved plaque control. It is the patient who has the essential role here. It is therefore important to understand the subject of patient motivation and behaviour change before offering any preventive advice. The preventive treatment required should be planned by the dentist who may delegate some tasks to a therapist, a hygienist, or a

---

FACTORS THAT INFLUENCE COMPLIANCE[1]

- Compliance with healthcare advice tends to be poor in patients who have non-life-threatening chronic conditions such as dental caries.

- Patients with good levels of oral hygiene tend to comply better with advice than those whose initial plaque levels are high.

- The patient's perception of their degree of control over what happens to them may be relevant. Those who believe what happens depends on their own behaviour (a high **internal locus of control**) may do better than those who believe what happens depends on luck, fate, or professional intervention (a high **external locus of control**).

- Socio-economic status is related to health behaviour, with less compliance from lower socio-economic groups.

- An unwillingness to perform self-care, a poor understanding of the problem and stressful life events may all be associated with poor compliance.

- Oral health behaviour is linked to other healthy lifestyle habits such as not smoking, taking exercise, and a healthy diet.

dental health educator. In this chapter the operator is often referred to as 'the dentist', but the information is applicable to all members of the dental team.

8.2 DEFINITION OF MOTIVATION

To motivate is to stimulate the interest of a person, causing them to act. There has been much misunderstanding surrounding patient motivation and it has often erroneously been thought of as either simply telling a patient what to do and telling them again if they have not complied the first time, or as a simple technique of forcing them to change their behaviour. Motivation is about creating the desire within another to want to follow advice for their own benefit. Good communication is the foundation for motivation. Compliance is not likely where patients do not understand, or cannot remember, the message.

8.3 COMMUNICATION

There is a tendency to think that because we learn to speak from an early age (and on average we each use up to 5000 words per day), communication is not a skill that can be learnt or improved upon once we become adults. Just as the ability to do operative dentistry is learnt, practiced, and perfected, so it is with communication skills.

The work of Mehrabian[2] suggests that communication is made up of three parts:
- 7% actual words conveying information
- 38% tone conveying emotions and attitudes
- 55% non-verbal communication also conveying emotions and attitudes.

Understanding the relative importance of these components may explain why communication sometimes breaks down and why patients often appear unmotivated and non-compliant. These components will now be considered in more detail.

8.3.1 Actual words

The following factors can affect the success of communication in the verbal channel:

Use of open and closed questions

Open questions allow the patient a free possibility of response and encourage the patient to discuss all their concerns. These questions initiate discussion and closed questions may then focus down on the issues as the patient raises them. To give examples: 'is anything worrying you about your mouth?' is an open question, whereas, 'are you concerned about the number of fillings I suggest?' is a closed question.

Dental jargon

Patients frequently misunderstand common dental words. The patient may have frequently heard the words 'plaque', 'caries', and 'bacteria', but may not know their real meaning. Information should be given simply and it is not unreasonable to check a patient's understanding by asking a question such as 'Can you tell me what you understand by the term plaque?' Some patients think plaque is calculus, and therefore the dentist's responsibility to remove and not theirs.

Words chosen in giving explanations will vary according to the knowledge and expectations of the listener. The listener should be neither belittled nor befuddled by the message. Explaining the cause of caries to a chemistry graduate will differ from the explanation offered to a child.

Listening and empathy

Research suggests that we only listen at 25% of our full potential. The patient may be anxious about dental treatment or have other pressing things on the mind such as collecting the children from school or an important business meeting. Thus information given is not always received, remembered, or acted upon.

To overcome this, advice and instructions should be given early in an appointment with the most important point being stressed, and then repeated or summarized as the patient leaves the surgery. If the instructions are also written down, the patient has less chance of forgetting or distorting what was agreed. The dentist's message to a caries-prone patient at the beginning of the appointment may be 'To prevent further holes in your teeth it is going to be very important for you to reduce the number of sugar "attacks" you have each day.' This can be restated as the patient leaves the surgery as 'So we've agreed the most important thing you are going to do is to try an artificial sweetener in your tea and coffee to cut down the sugar "attacks".'

It is important that the dentist listens to what the patient has to say. We are also guilty of listening with only a half or even a quarter of an ear to our patients. Empathy refers to the feeling that the listener is making an effort to understand the situation from the speaker's point of view. Perhaps a patient talks about the difficulty of finding time or energy at the end of the day for an oral hygiene routine. The professional can now discuss the time taken and how this can be fitted into the patient's lifestyle.

Forgetting

Patients forget advice more than other types of information and it is suggested that 50% of information given is forgotten within 5 minutes of a patient leaving the surgery.[3] It is important not to overload the patient with information, as three or four key points are the most they are likely to remember at one appointment.

Distortion

There is a tendency to distort what we have heard and to put our own interpretation on it. Patients taught the Bass technique of brushing may return brushing vigorously using the 'up and down' technique, believing they are following the dentist's advice. Dietary advice also gets distorted. A 12-year-old girl with a high caries rate was advised to stop drinking squash containing sugar and to buy sugar-free squash instead. Her father, who brought her for her dental appointment, agreed that they would do this. Written instructions were given to the parents. A subsequent phone conversation with the girl's mother some weeks later elicited that they had purchased a 'reduced sugar' squash which unfortunately was also cariogenic.

8.3.2 Tone

Tone conveys attitudes and emotions such as enthusiasm or boredom. Patients will soon detect these emotions from the dentist's tone of voice and while enthusiasm is infectious, boredom is demotivating. Dentists can also detect a patient's emotions from the tone of their voice. When this tone indicates a message has not been well received it is worth trying to discuss the matter further. A comment from the dentist such as 'I don't think I've convinced you', may open the door to exploring the perceived difficulty with the patient.

8.3.3 Non-verbal communication or body language

Facial expression

One of the main functions of facial expression is to communicate emotions and attitudes, and it may be that a dentist will know a patient has no intention of following advice given just by observing the patient's facial expression. The patient will also pick up the facial expression of the dentist, which may inadvertently register judgement, disapproval, disbelief, or even dislike. This can affect communication and ultimately motivation. Conversely, facial expression can be used to enhance motivation. Something as simple as a smile helps to put patients at their ease and enhance trust. In a particularly unpleasant experiment the facial muscles of some infant monkeys and their mothers were cut and it was found that the pairs failed to develop any relationship with each other.

Eye contact

Eye contact is important because it enables both the dentist and the patient to collect information which can be used to guide the way the consultation is going. Students report feeling very frustrated when patients gaze out of the window while they are talking to them and will not give them eye contact. They say 'I've no idea if they are listening to me or not—I don't know whether to go on or to stop'. When advice is being offered, ensure that the patient is seated at the same level as you are and not lying supine. If the patient continues to avoid eye contact, stop talking and wait to see what effect this has. If this fails, acknowledge that the patient does not appear to be listening and say 'You seem uninterested in what I am saying. Is there a reason for this?' This should bring eye contact back and provide the opportunity for the patient to explain what they are finding difficult.

To know how it feels to be a patient, try lying in the dental chair, and attempt to floss or brush watching yourself in a mirror held by a colleague who is also giving you advice. All eye contact is lost and there is a sense of being 'talked down to' and a strong feeling of disempowerment.

Gestures and bodily movements

When emotions are aroused, pointless bodily movements are often made. For example, an anxious patient may scratch their neck or adjust their jacket or skirt. A patient unwilling to state that they have not used the fluoride mouthwash recommended at the last visit may, for example, brush imaginary fluff from their sleeve when asked about mouthwash use.

Bodily posture

Posture can communicate as clearly as words. If the dentist is running late, and the patient in the waiting room is standing with their hands on their hips and chin thrust forward, this communicates a warning to 'proceed with caution!' When running late it is wise to inform the patient of the delay and apologize for it. Starting with an immediate apology will usually defuse a potentially explosive situation.

Bodily contact

Bodily contact in our culture is controlled by strict rules and is used mainly by families and courting couples. Professionals such as doctors and dentists use it, but not as a social act. In dentistry the adult patient usually accepts without question that their visit will involve touch, but it should be remembered that bodily contact can also help or hinder communication. A firm handshake in greeting may increase a patient's confidence in their dentist, but not all students feel comfortable doing this or indeed think that it is always necessary or appropriate. A hand on the shoulder of an anxious patient as the dental chair is taken back may convey care for the patient and be reassuring to those who are anxious, but a confident patient may feel patronized or annoyed by it. Each case needs to be assessed individually.

Spatial behaviour

In most walks of life the importance of personal space is recognized and respected, apart from situations where overcrowding is accepted as normal, such as lifts and crowded public transport. Four spatial zones have been suggested:

- intimate zone   15–50 cm
- personal zone   50 cm–1.2 m
- social zone   1.2–3.6 m
- public zone   3.6 m

The personal space referred to as the 'intimate zone' is usually reserved for close friends, but it is automatically invaded when a dentist examines or operates. This is accepted by patients, but it is worth remembering that for some patients there maybe some embarrassment and anxiety that affects them receiving the dentist's communication in this 'intimate zone'. Just because it is culturally acceptable, it should not be taken to be without meaning for the patient.[4] When giving advice to a patient it is a good idea to return the dental chair to the upright position, ensure that eye contact is on the same level and move away from the patient to a position where communication is comfortable for both parties.

Clothes and appearance

Clothes and appearance communicate information. For example, a white coat may communicate one thing to a patient whereas a blue or green coat may communicate something different. One study showed that children's heart rates increased by 10 beats per minute when a dentist put on a white coat.[5] Badges too communicate information. The paediatric dentist who wears a teddy bear badge is communicating a message to a child patient and to the parent.

The style and décor of the surgery and waiting room also communicate a message to patients. Dental students who were asked to rate the skill and competence of several hypothetical dentists by looking at photographs of old fashioned, modern, and ultra-modern surgeries, inferred that a dentist with an ultra-modern surgery would be more trustworthy, more skilful, and more competent. Something as simple as plants, lighting, types and states of magazines all communicate, albeit at a subconscious level. One patient, when asked what she thought of the dentist's waiting room, pointed to the posters on the walls displaying pictures of bad gums and teeth and said 'Tell the dentist to take those home and put them on his sitting room wall and bring us in the pictures he's got hanging there instead'.

8.4 FACTORS THAT ENHANCE LEARNING

Once patients have received information it is important that they remember it. Here are some specific suggestions to help patients remember advice.

8.4.1 Involving the patient

When the dentist hopes to motivate a patient to remember and comply with health advice it is not enough just to tell them or show them, there is also a need to involve them. This can be done in the surgery in a number of ways such as:

- asking the patient to brush or floss during oral hygiene instruction
- showing them an extracted decayed tooth or their own radiograph
- encouraging them to feel a piece of calculus you have removed from their teeth
- offering them a sugar-free mint to taste
- asking them to take away and complete a diet analysis sheet.

8.4.2 Making use of other senses

There is a tendency to rely only on verbal communication forgetting that sight, sound, touch, taste, and smell can all be used. More may be remembered if more than one sense is used to receive information. Thus involving a patient's senses of sight, hearing, and touch in learning anything new is likely to bring about a greater retention of material than if only one of these senses is used.

It is not difficult to involve senses other than hearing. For instance when teaching patients to use a toothbrush the dentist may place a hand over the patient's hand to guide their movement. The patient will **feel** the brush touching the gingivae and **hear** how little noise is made by the brush when the Bass technique is correctly carried out. Ineffective scrubbing with a brush is noisy, but effective insertion of the filaments interdentally and vibratory movement is quiet. The patient may also **see** blood on the filaments. It is important to explain that this is a consequence of inflammation and does not imply the patient has been rough. Finally, the patient can be encouraged to run their tongue over the teeth to **feel** the shiny, smooth surface of plaque-free teeth. Similarly, the senses can be used when teaching a patient to floss. The patient may be able to **see** plaque on the floss, **smell** the putrid odour of plaque removed from a stagnation area, and **feel** calculus obstructing free movement of the floss.

8.4.3 Amount of information given

Patients are unlikely to remember more than three or four key points at any one appointment. The important points should be made first and emphasized. It is sensible to give less information rather than more and check that it has been understood. Many patients, either wishing to please or trying to avoid looking foolish, will nod readily when listening to advice being given but often have not really understood. Sometimes understanding can be checked. For instance if a fluoride mouthwash has been recommended, at the end of the appointment the patient could be asked to use it. This is not to 'catch the patient out' but to help the dentist see if the message given earlier has been understood and give help if necessary.

8.4.4 Short, simple, and specific advice

Most of us find it difficult to remember complex and lengthy explanations of subjects which are not our particular speciality. Advice to patients has a greater chance of being retained and acted upon if it is kept short, simple, and specific. So to say to a patient with white spot lesions 'You have several white spot lesions and early areas of demineralization which may respond to a regime of fluoride therapy', would not be helpful. Saying 'There are lots of new holes starting in your teeth. I would like you to use a fluoride mouthwash daily to try to prevent them from getting any worse' gets the message home simply and clearly.

8.4.5 Timing

Timing of preventive advice is important. For example, it will not be well received by a patient in pain. However, once toothache has been relieved preventive treatment may be accepted as relevant to prevent recurrence of the problem.

Preventive advice should not be relegated to the end of an appointment because the patient may be tired and anxious to leave. Operative and preventive treatment may be combined in one appointment, but the preventive element requires maximum patient participation and should be carried out first. Some preventive items take longer than others. The time for a local anaesthetic to work may be sufficient to show a patient how to use a mouthwash. Dietary analysis and advice is more time consuming and may require a separate appointment.

It is surprising how often students will scale a quadrant and then give oral hygiene instruction. This is illogical, since the plaque that the patient should see will have been removed. Oral hygiene instruction should precede scaling. However, even this rule is made to be broken sometimes. It may be helpful for a patient with very heavy plaque and calculus deposits to have one quadrant professionally cleaned before oral hygiene instruction so that they can see and feel the difference this has made.

Social history is often relevant to the timing of preventive treatment. For instance, flossing is time consuming. When does the patient have the time to do this? It is sensible to discuss this and let the patient suggest the appropriate time. Flossing is also somewhat tedious and it may be helpful to link the behaviour with something else, e.g. flossing while taking a bath, listening to music.

8.4.6 A telephone reminder

A telephone call to discuss progress, remind the patient, and support their efforts can be helpful. It can be particularly useful to remind a patient of their appointment and to remember to bring something essential (e.g. a completed diet sheet) to the surgery.

8.5 FACTORS AFFECTING MOTIVATION

Sometimes clear communication of a dental health message results in behaviour change which is apparent by a change in oral health. To give an example, a patient with inflamed gums is shown a new cleaning technique; gingival inflammation subsides and health is restored. This is very satisfying for all concerned but it does not always happen. Let us say that in the same circumstances, the patient returns with the same gingival inflammation and the same heavy plaque deposits. When this happens the following factors are worth considering.

8.5.1 Diagnosing the problem; skill or motivation?

The dentist needs to diagnose the problem. Perhaps the patient has not understood the message or, because they are insufficiently skilled, they cannot achieve what was asked. This diagnosis can be straightforward. If plaque is disclosed the dentist can discover whether the patient can remove it. If they **can**, but **do not**, the problem is one of motivation.

Changing a patient's knowledge does not necessarily change their behaviour. Smoking is an excellent example of this. Many smokers know the adverse effects of cigarettes but choose to ignore them.

8.5.2 Whose problem?

Many people are ignorant about dental disease and do not recognize it as a problem. This is partly an indictment of our role as educators. Many patients think that it is the dentist's responsibility to care for their mouths. However, in a year a dentist may see a patient for less than 1 hour out of the total 8760. Since plaque continually reforms, its removal has to be the responsibility of the patient. It is vital that patients recognize and acknowledge this and therefore the dental team must take time to talk and listen to them.

Many people have grown up with the idea that it is inevitable and normal to need fillings and even lose teeth. A middle-aged patient, on being told he had five new holes in his teeth remarked 'Well that's not bad, is it—after all I am 45, so I've done pretty well to have kept my teeth as long as this, haven't I?' Such a patient is accepting and unconcerned about ongoing disease in his mouth. Attempts at motivation stand a greater chance of success if the dentist first shares his or her concern and then finds out what level of concern, if any, the patient has. This is an important starting place and will guide the dentist as to how to proceed. It will prevent premature and apparently irrelevant advice being given.

8.5.3 Patients' beliefs

It must not be taken for granted that a patient holds the same beliefs as the dentist. This is illustrated by the following case. A middle-aged executive secretary attended with a very heavily restored mouth and multiple carious lesions around restorations. Although her oral hygiene was reasonable, her diet was very unfavourable as the patient continually worked with sugared tea or coffee on her desk. This patient's father had been a dentist and she was brought up to believe he could cope with anything by using the drill. Unfortunately this was no longer possible, as there was insufficient tooth tissue left to restore.

It is important to take time to find out what patients believe, because this will affect the advice given and subsequently compliance. In this case time and effort was spent attempting to modify the patient's beliefs, but this was a failure. The patient politely declined further appointments and sought a new dentist who would 'treat her', by which she meant 'fill her teeth.'

8.5.4 Personally relevant advice

If patients are to change their behaviour they must see the advice offered as being relevant to them. It is easy to give every patient the same advice, such as how to brush and floss, the importance of dietary control of sugar, and use of a fluoride mouthwash. However, it is important that the advice is tailored to the individual needs of the patient. For example, there is no point in persuading a 50-year-old-patient to complete a diet analysis sheet if examination reveals that caries is not a current problem.

8.5.5 Enthusiasm

A salesperson who strongly believes in the product engenders enthusiasm and interest in the potential purchaser. 'Selling' the concept of dental health to a patient has a greater chance of success if the dentist promotes 'the product' with enthusiasm. Words such as 'This small-headed brush will really help you to get to those back teeth and you'll notice they no longer feel furred up but shiny and clean' encourage a patient to feel spending extra time on plaque removal is worthwhile.

8.5.6 High trust—low fear

Trust between dentist and patient often develops over time. It is in a high-trust environment that patients are more likely to follow advice, so it is important to continue to develop a good relationship so that trust increases with each visit. The response that the dentist hopes for may take several years of patience and understanding.

When patients are slow to follow advice, it may be tempting to resort to threatening them with the consequence. Studies[6] have shown that while the use of fear and threat may produce behaviour change, this is limited to the short term. Fear and threat should therefore be used cautiously. 'I am concerned about the number of new cavities you have in your teeth' may be a much better approach then 'If you don't follow my advice you are going to lose all your teeth by the time you are 60!'

8.5.7 Care

If the dentist can convey to the patient that they care about them and have a genuine interest in their dental health, compliance is more likely. Thus, to say to a patient who is struggling with dental floss 'It looks as though you find that extremely awkward to use' lets the patient know you understand their difficulties. The dentist can then offer alternatives, such as bottle brushes, which the patient may find easier to use.

8.5.8 Praise

Praise is a strong motivator and patients respond positively to this, whereas rebuke demotivates them. One patient was heard to remark that he gave up trying to brush better because no matter how hard he tried, his efforts were constantly criticized. Even if there is only a slight improvement or a small change in behaviour it is important to acknowledge this in a positive way. This can be done by saying 'I can see you have put a lot of effort into your brushing and the gums look very much better around your front teeth'. After this, further advice can be offered in the areas where there is still room for improvement.

8.5.9 Negotiation

Szasz and Hollender[7] state that there are three types of relationship that may exist between patients and health professionals:
- **The active–passive relationship** where the dentist assumes total responsibility for the patient who remains passive in the encounter. A patient having a general anaesthetic would be an example of this.
- **The guidance–cooperation relationship** where the dentist is seen as the 'expert' who gives advice with which the patient is expected to comply.

- **The mutual participation relationship** where the dentist and the patient share equally. The patient's thoughts, ideas, and beliefs are considered as important as the dentist's advice and technical expertise. This relationship is the most appropriate to motivate patients to adopt preventive health behaviours. Thus there is a greater chance of a patient following health advice if negotiation has taken place.

For example, if the dentist feels the patient should cut our sugar in drinks and use an artificial sweetener instead, it would be best to negotiate with the patient rather than dictate to them. A question such as 'How would you feel about trying to give up sugar in tea and coffee?' or 'What would you feel about trying an artificial sweetener?' would be ways of negotiating with a patient. This provides them with the opportunity to share their beliefs or ideas which are important because these attitudes affect compliance.

On being asked to try an artificial sweetener in tea or coffee, patients will often comment that they do not like the taste of artificial sweeteners and would therefore find it hard to change their habits. In this situation, it may be helpful to make a number of cups of tea or coffee for the patient sweetened with various artificial sweeteners and one cup sweetened with sugar. Each cup should be designated by a letter and the patient asked to rank the acceptability of the drink with marks out of 10. Surprisingly, some patients cannot recognize sugar and will give one of the artificial sweeteners an equal ranking. This demonstration can aid the negotiation and be a powerful motivating tool, encouraging the patient to buy the appropriate sugar substitute.

8.5.10 Realistic goals

With an enthusiastic approach to motivation it is easy to set a patient unrealistic goals without appreciating their point of view. For example, a patient who is told to brush for half an hour a day will not comply with this advice because it is totally unrealistic. If the patient is included in the negotiation (see section 8.5.9) it is likely that a realistic goal with be set. For instance if a dentist would like a patient to floss, the importance of flossing should be discussed and the technique demonstrated in one part of the mouth, perhaps on an approximal surface where an enamel lesion is present on radiograph. The patient can be asked how often it would be realistic to floss this contact. If the patient suggests flossing the area twice a week, this should be accepted as a realistic goal. In learning any new skill it is important to build in small steps. At subsequent visits, dentist and patient may together decide to move the goal posts, perhaps by agreeing to floss the same area daily or by including other susceptible contact points.

8.5.11 Regular positive reinforcement and follow-up

Maintaining changes in behaviour in the long term is difficult. Broken New Year resolutions are an obvious example. It is therefore important that a patient's progress is followed up regularly, and positive reinforcement offered where they have maintained changes in their behaviour. For example, where agreement to try an artificial sweetener in place of sugar was reached on the first appointment, an opening gambit on the second appointment could be 'How have you got on with the artificial sweetener?' At a 3-month review appointment the patient should be asked whether the artificial sweetener is still being used. This encourages the patient to maintain the change.

For the dentist to be able to check how the patient is progressing on subsequent appointments it is important that the notes are fully written up after each visit so that they can be referred to before the next appointment. The notes may say for example:

Patient has agreed to:
- Buy fluoride mouthrinse and use daily
- Floss contact between LL5 and LL6 twice a week
- Complete diet sheet and return it next visit

These agreed goals should also be written down at the end of the appointment for the patient to take away because it is easy to forget or misinterpret what was agreed. The notes also provide the dentist with a good starting point on the next visit. 'Did you manage to buy the fluoride mouthwash after your last visit?' and also provide the opportunity to offer positive reinforcement to encourage the patient.

A record can also be kept of any aspect of the patient's social history that may be useful. A patient was amazed and pleased when his dentist asked at a 6-month follow-up appointment 'Have you started outdoor bowls yet this year?' The patient commented what an excellent memory the dentist had. In fact it was because the dentist **hadn't** got a good memory that he had made a note of the patient's hobby. Comments such as these can help to build relationships with patients and may enhance motivation.

8.5.12 Scoring

A scoring system that enables both dentist and patient to monitor behaviour change may be helpful. For instance a simple system of scoring plaque may be used. If the patient is told that an acceptable plaque score is around 10% and after disclosing he or she learns that the score is a lot higher than this, the effect can be to encourage further effort. At the next appointment the patient's opening remarks are often 'What's my score today? I've worked hard at trying to get it down since I last saw you.

USEFUL STEPS TOWARDS BEHAVIOUR CHANGE

- Specify the goals that the dental team and the patient wish to achieve
- Plan the specific behaviour change
- Decide when to start
- Provide opportunities to practice the new behaviour and perfect technique
- Advise those close to the patient about the change and seek their support
- Decide when and how the change will occur
- Build in rewards for success
- Review progress and rectify problems

8.6 PLANNING BEHAVIOUR CHANGE[8]

Behaviour change can be difficult to achieve, and planning may be helpful (see box).

The following case illustrates some of these points. A young woman brought her fiancé to the dentist. His oral hygiene was poor, the gingivae were inflamed and there were multiple white spot lesions. Diet analysis showed an eating pattern of fast foods, sweet fizzy drinks, sugary snacks, and very little fruit or vegetables.

The couple wanted the young man's mouth to look good in the wedding photographs. The matter was urgent: a wedding in 3 months' time. The dentist wanted to improve both oral hygiene and diet.

An immediate start was made with oral hygiene instruction showing both of them what needed to be done and explaining to them how the appearance of the gums should change with cleaning from red, swollen, and bleeding to pink and firm.

Dietary changes were discussed. The woman decided to make a packed lunch (more fruit, bottled water) and said she would stop buying sweet fizzy drinks so they were just not available. She also commented that on the new regime, **she** would lose weight and also look better in the wedding photographs.

The couple continued to come to see the oral health educator every 3 weeks, and although progress with improving cleaning was slow, it was sure. The wedding photographs were proudly brought to the surgery.

The sting in the tail of the story is that once the wedding was over, oral hygiene regressed (but not to its original low level) and the patient started to miss appointments.

8.7 REVIEWING PROGRESS AND RECTIFYING PROBLEMS

In the case described above, regular reviews were important. The common problems that occur in behaviour change are:
- skills deficits
- the goal is too difficult
- the consequences of the behaviour are too far removed
- 'forgetting'.

In the case discussed above the man had some trouble mastering the new oral hygiene regime. He brushed well, but not for long enough. As a night shift worker, he found time was a problem, as was energy at the end of a shift. The consequence of the altered behaviour, a nice smile on the wedding photograph, was imminent but once this motivation had gone, it was not easy to keep up the new behaviour pattern. When he was tired he would forget to brush so his wife, at the dentist's suggestion, put a tick chart in the bathroom and checked it was completed.

8.8 FAILURE

It would be nice to think that if all the advice in this chapter was followed, failures in patient motivation would never occur. This is not the case. One third to one half of all patients fail to follow fully the advice given to them. This may be for all manner of reasons, many of which have been discussed in this chapter. If you feel you have failed to motivate a patient it is worth asking yourself, in the light of the contents of this chapter, if there is anything you could or should have done differently.

Some psychological theories may throw additional light on issues of non-compliance.
- The **health belief model**[9] states that for an individual to take action they have to believe they are susceptible to the disease, that the disease is serious, and the benefits of following the prescribed advice outweigh the costs. Many patients may not believe caries is serious or that they are susceptible to it. For some patients the cost of spending extra time in the bathroom flossing and rinsing with a fluoride mouthwash outweighs any perceived benefit and this may explain why they have not followed the advice given.
- The **health locus of control theory**[9] states that individuals hold beliefs about whether they have any control over what happens to them. They may have a fatalistic approach: 'Teeth just rot; there's nothing I can do about it.' This demonstrates an external locus of control where the patient believes fate or chance are in control. They may say 'It's the dentist's responsibility to care for my mouth, not mine' demonstrating an external

locus of control where the patient believes 'powerful others' are in control of what happens. Conversely, they may have an internal locus of control and say 'I believe I can prevent further holes in my teeth'. The latter patient will not be hard to motivate but the two former examples will need all the educator's enthusiasm, patience, and skill.

- The **theory of reasoned action**[10] states that an individual will only perform a certain behaviour if they perceive it is worthwhile and if others who are significant to them also believe the same thing. Thus a teenage patient who the dentist tries to persuade to attend for regular check-ups may not comply because they are influenced by their peer group who do not believe regular dental attendance is worthwhile. Similarly, a patient whose family members have false teeth with which they are quite happy may not listen to the attempts of the educator to persuade them to give up sugar in drinks in order to prevent them from finishing up with false teeth.

The importance of the dental team should not be underestimated in patient motivation. What the dentist may not be able to achieve, the hygienist, nurse, or dental health educator may, or vice versa. Sometimes it can be something as simple as a different personality taking over which changes the outcome.

Motivation of patients can be a slow process. It does not usually happen after one visit. It is often a continuous process of building up trust and rapport with a patient over many visits, continuing to be encouraging and finding small improvements that the educator can be positive about. It is also an ethical necessity to be honest with patients, and there will be times when we will have to confront the patient and tell them their preventive efforts are insufficient to prevent dental disease.

As dental health educators we need to remember we can lead a horse to water, but we can't make it drink. Ours is the business of creating the environment that makes the 'horse' thirsty.

Further reading and references

1. Ower, P. (2003) The role of self administered plaque control in the management of periodontal diseases: 2. Motivation, techniques and assessment. *Dent. Update*, **30**, 110–116.
2. Mehrabian, A. (1971) *Silent messages*. Wadsworth, Belmont, CA.
3. Ley, P., Bradshaw, P. W., Eaves, D., and Walker, C. M. (1973) A method for increasing patients' recall of information presented by doctors. *Psychol. Med.*, **3**, 217–220.
4. Kent, G. and Croucher, R. (1998) *Achieving oral health. The social context of dental care*. Wright, Oxford.
5. Simpson, W. J., Ruzicka, R. L., and Thomas N. R. (1974) Physiologic responses to initial dental experience. *J. Dent. Child.*, **41**, 465–470.
6. Janis, I. L. and Feshbach, S. (1953) Effect of fear-arousing communications. *J. Abnorm. Psychol.*, **48**, 78.
7. Szasz, T. S. and Hollender, M. H. (1956) A contribution to the philosophy of medicine: the basic models of the doctor-patient relationship. *Arch. Intern. Med.*, **97**, 585–592.

8. Palmer, R. and Floyd, P. (2002) *Guide to periodontology*. Ch.4: Patient motivation and communication. BDJ Books, London.

9. Weinman, J. (1987) *An outline of psychology as applied to medicine*. Wright, Bristol.

10. Broome, A. (ed.) (1989) *Health psychology: processes and application*. Ch.1: Health beliefs and attributions. Chapman & Hall, London.

9

The operative management of caries

9.1 THE ROLE OF OPERATIVE TREATMENT IN CARIES MANAGEMENT

9.1.1 What constitutes treatment?

Practising dentists spend a major part of their time, and derive a substantial part of their income, from repairing the ravages of dental caries. Restorative dentistry is technically demanding, and dental schools must devote many curriculum hours to this subject so that graduates are technically competent. Unfortunately, this emphasis, although essential, has its dangers. The undergraduate may come to believe that operative dentistry **is** the treatment of the carious process. However, as explained on page 3, the carious process occurs in the biofilm and its reflection is the lesion in the tooth. To concentrate only on a reflection, to the exclusion of the cause, would be ridiculous.

Dental schools may have reinforced this attitude by operating 'points systems' where points were given for operative procedures and students were signed up to take their final examination once a certain number of points had been achieved. Points were not usually awarded for preventive treatments and thus undergraduates felt that to be working, they must be restoring teeth.

These attitudes were perhaps also fuelled by the method of remuneration of dentists in the UK National Health Service. For many years dentists were paid a fee per item of reparative treatment but preventive treatments, such as dietary advice, fluoride application, oral hygiene instructions, and fissure sealing, were not individually remunerated. These attitudes were inevitably transferred to patients. Students or dentists who spend time on preventive treatments were asked by patients, 'When are you going to do something?', meaning 'When are you going to place a filling?' Thus over the years treatment of caries in adults become synonymous with operative dentistry and prevention was designated as 'the wait and watch' approach, implying inactivity. On the other hand, departments of children's dentistry were more enlightened.

Dental schools now teach cariology together with operative dentistry so that students can appreciate that the carious process can be modified by preventive treatment. Chapters 4–8 of this text have concentrated on these treatment techniques. They are the essential management of the carious process and are time-consuming and therefore expensive, although cost-effective in the long run. The techniques are just as worthy of remuneration as operative dentistry. Thus treatment of the carious process involves both preventive treatment and operative treatment.

Since preventive treatments demand the full cooperation of the patient, it is extremely important that patients appreciate that appointments addressing plaque control, dietary advice, and use of fluoride are just as much

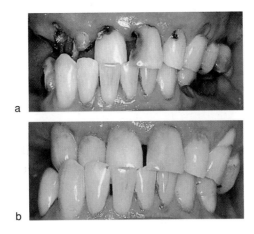

Figure 9.1. Before (a) and after (b), a course of treatment by an undergraduate dental student. This patient presented with a very neglected mouth and with poor motivation and low expectations of treatment. However, he has not only benefited from the student's operative treatment but also heeded the preventive advice and encouragement given. He is now highly motivated towards his remaining teeth and his whole attitude to dentistry has been changed by this experience.

treatment of the carious process as appointments to place restorations. Indeed, since few of us actually like having our teeth filled, a dentist whose philosophy is to help patients avoid the need for fillings will be popular!

However, high-risk patients often present requiring restorations. The dentist may find it more difficult to explain the importance of preventive treatment when the patient is experiencing discomfort and/or a cosmetic problem (Figure 9.1a). In these cases treating the patient's problem (such as pain or an unsightly filling) is very important if the dentist is going to gain the patient's trust and cooperation in future preventive management. When discussing the importance of preventive treatment with a patient, a useful analogy can be drawn with the problem presented by a building that is on fire. It would be illogical to repair the building before the flames were extinguished.

9.1.2 Why treat operatively?

The most important reason for placing a restoration is to aid plaque control. If a patient is unable to clean plaque out of a hole in a tooth, the carious process is almost bound to progress.

The other reasons for recommending restorative treatment are:[1]
- The tooth is sensitive to hot, cold and sweet. Dentine is a good insulator but when a tooth is cavitated some of this insulation is lost. Sensitivity is less likely in chronic lesions where tubular sclerosis and tertiary dentine have reduced dentine permeability.

- The pulp is endangered (see page 33).
- Previous attempts to arrest the lesion have failed and there is evidence the lesion is progressing (this usually requires an observation period of months or years).
- Function is impaired.
- Drifting is likely to occur through loss of a contact point.
- For aesthetic reasons. The cosmetic improvement can be very satisfying and the dentist will enjoy restoring teeth, smiles, function and dental health (Figure 9.1).

9.1.3 When to treat operatively[2]

The anatomy of the **fissure** can favour plaque stagnation and this is particularly likely during eruption of the tooth[3] (see page 74). When an active enamel lesion is diagnosed in a fissure, or if a high risk is established and fissures are sound, a **fissure sealant** could be indicated.[4] This resin coat, physically attached to the enamel via the acid etch technique, prevents plaque accumulation on an occlusal surface. Sealants are safe and effective in preventing caries in susceptible teeth and individuals, provided the sealant remains in place.[5]

The technique does not involve cutting the tooth, and active lesions covered by the resin do not progress further. Where sealants are placed over dentine caries, there is ample evidence that lesions do not progress provided the sealant remains in place.[2]

Cavitated occlusal lesions require **restorations** because the shape of the cavity (Figure 2.10) precludes plaque control.

Where a cavitated carious lesion is present on an **approximal** surface, the adjacent tooth may prevent plaque removal and the lesion is likely to progress. Referring to the radiographic appearance of approximal caries (Figure 3.10), R4 lesions are always cavitated and should be treated operatively. R3 lesions may or may not be cavitated. Cavitation is more likely in a high-risk patient. Separating the teeth will allow an accurate diagnosis (see page 54).

Cavities on **free smooth surfaces** are often easily reached by a toothbrush. However, where the process is undermining the enamel, removal of the overhanging enamel margins by grinding and polishing should be considered to aid cleaning (Figure 9.2). These cavities, be they on enamel or root surfaces, can be arrested and converted to hard lesions over a period of months by twice daily cleaning with a fluoride toothpaste.

This approach does not always work because the quality of plaque removal is crucial for arresting active carious lesions. Where the approach is not working, where the patient cannot access the plaque, or where the cavity is unsightly, restorations are indicated (Figure 9.3). Even when oral hygiene is inadequate, placing a restoration gives the patient **time to improve** by

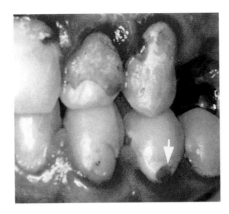

Figure 9.2. This patient presented with a very neglected mouth; poor oral hygiene, a high-sugar diet and several carious lesions. Before this picture was taken, a disclosing agent was used and the patient was shown how to brush off the plaque. The buccal cavity in the lower premolar is plaque free except where enamel is overhanging the lesion. Removal of this enamel would make it easier to arrest the lesion by plaque control alone.

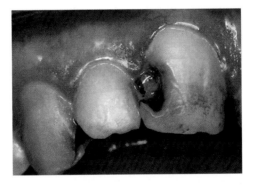

Figure 9.3. The patient finds this lesion difficult to clean and it is unsightly. A restoration is indicated, but the patient should be taught to keep the margins of the filling clean otherwise a new lesion will form next to the filling.

sending the carious process (the metabolic activity in the plaque) back to the tooth surface to start again. It's a dental version of Snakes and Ladders.

9.2 FISSURE SEALING

9.2.1 Isolation

Isolation is probably the most critical step with regard to the success or failure of the sealant. If saliva blocks the pores created by etching, the bond

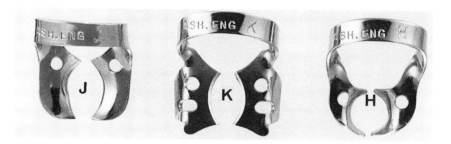

Figure 9.4. A selection of rubber dam clamps. Clamps J and K are bland, H is retentive, J and H are wingless, K is winged.

will be weakened. A rubber dam is the most effective method of isolation and is preferred to the use of cotton-wool rolls and a saliva ejector. The latter are difficult to use, because after etching the teeth must be thoroughly washed. This inevitably soaks the cotton-wool rolls, which must then be changed. While this is being done, it is all too easy to drop saliva over the etched tooth surface and this contamination will ruin the bond of the sealant to the enamel. When a rubber dam is applied for fissure sealing, only the tooth to be treated needs to be isolated. Since a rubber dam clamp will be required, and clamps can be uncomfortable, a small amount of local anaesthetic should be infiltrated buccal to the tooth to be treated. Alternatively, topical anaesthetic may be liberally applied to the gingival margin. A clamp of suitable size is selected and tried on the tooth, placing it just coronal to the gingival margin. Where the maximum convexity of the tooth is subgingival, a retentive rubber dam clamp is required, but where the tooth is fully erupted, a bland clamp should be chosen (see Figure 9.4). Floss should be attached to the holes of the clamp so that the dentist can retrieve it should the clamp fracture across the bow (Figure 9.5a).

If the clamp is positioned before applying the rubber, it is convenient to select a wingless clamp for molar teeth (Figure 9.5a). Having placed the clamp on the tooth, the floss is threaded through the punched and lubricated hole in the rubber dam (Figure 9.5b). The dental nurse now gently pulls on the floss as the dentist slides the rubber over the bow of the clamp, one side (Figure 9.5c) and then the other side. Should the clamp fracture across the bow, the dental nurse retrieves the pieces by pulling on the floss.

An alternative technique is for the dentist to apply clamp and rubber simultaneously. In this case a winged clamp must be chosen (see Figure 9.4) and the wings engaged in the lubricated hole (Figure 9.6a). Clamp and rubber are applied simultaneously. The dental nurse assistant should gently retract the rubber so that the dentist can see the tooth clearly (Figure 9.6b). A disadvantage of this method is that the dentist cannot see the gingival margin when placing the clamp. Once the clamp is in position a flat plastic instrument is used to disengage the rubber from the wings of the clamp

(Figure 9.6c). If this step is omitted, saliva will leak around the tooth.

A piece of soft material, such as paper towelling, in which a mouth-hole has been cut, is now placed between the rubber and the patient's face to prevent the uncomfortable feeling of rubber against the face. Finally, the frame is positioned (Figure 9.7).

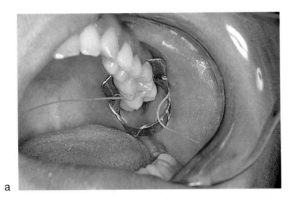

a

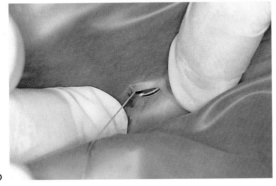

b

Figure 9.5. (a) A wingless clamp in position on an upper molar. Floss has been attached to the holes of the clamp so that the dentist can retrieve it should the clamp fracture across the bow. (b) The floss is now threaded through the punched and lubricated hole in the rubber dam. (c) The dentist now slides the rubber over the bow of the clamp, one side and then the other side. The dental nurse gently pulls on the floss as the rubber is placed.

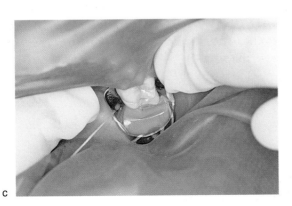

c

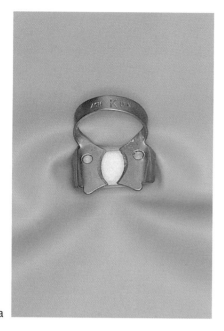

a

Figure 9.6. (a) A winged rubber dam clamp engaged in the hole in the rubber. (b) Clamp and rubber are being placed on the tooth simultaneously. The dental nurse should gently retract the rubber so that the dentist can see the tooth clearly. (c) A flat plastic instrument is used to disengage the rubber from the wings of the clamp.

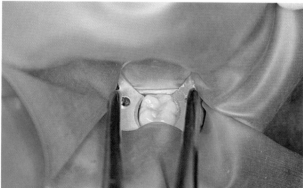

b

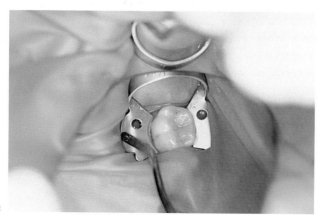

c

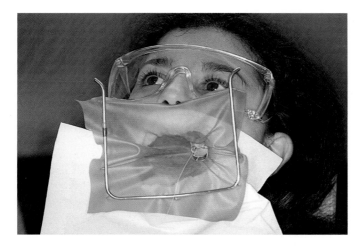

Figure 9.7. A rubber dam in position. Note that a soft paper towel separates the rubber from the face. The rubber may be trimmed to avoid contact with the nose, although this was not done in this case because the patient was comfortable.

9.2.2 Cleaning the teeth

The tooth surface to be etched and sealed must be thoroughly cleaned with a bristle brush and a pumice and water slurry. Oil-based mixtures of pumice should not be used as these may interfere with etching. The pumice is washed away with a blast of water and air from the three-in-one syringe and dried thoroughly.

9.2.3 Etching

The phosphoric acid etchant is supplied by the manufacturer in the form of either a liquid or a coloured gel. The gel is preferable as it is much easier to control. The etchant is applied over the whole occlusal surface and any lingual or buccal surface where grooves require sealing (Figure 9.8a). Etching the entire occlusal surface avoids the danger of covering an unetched surface with sealant and thus inviting leakage. The acid can be applied with either a tiny pledget of cotton wool, a tiny gauze sponge, or a small brush. As soon as the complete area to be etched is covered with acid, the time is noted. The etching time will be given in the manufacturer's instructions and is usually 30 seconds. When acid is used in the liquid form, fresh solution can be dabbed on the surface during etching but care should be taken to treat the enamel surface very carefully, and not rub the cotton pellet or sponge on the surface during acid application as this may damage the fragile enamel latticework being formed.

9.2.4 Washing

After etching, the acid is washed away. Initially a water spray is used from the three-in-one syringe to remove most of the acid. After approximately 5 seconds of spraying water, the air button is also pressed, forming a strong water–air spray which should be played over the etched surface for at least 15–20 seconds. If gels are used the wash time should be doubled to at least 30 seconds to ensure removal of the gel and reaction products. During the washing phase the dental nurse removes all excess water with the aspirator.

9.2.5 Drying the etched enamel

The tooth surface is now thoroughly dried with air from the three-in-one syringe. The drying phase is most important, since any moisture on the etched surface will hinder penetration of the resin into the enamel. A minimum of 15 seconds of drying is recommended. At this stage the etched area should appear matt and white (Figure 9.8b). It is good practice to check that the airline is not contaminated by water or oil by blowing it at a clean glass surface. Any moisture or oil coming from the airline will cause the technique to fail.

With a rubber dam in position, there should be no danger of salivary contamination of the etched surface. If this does occur, however, it is essential to re-etch the enamel because the saliva will block the pores which are essential for optimal bonding.

9.2.6 Mixing the resin

A light-cured resin material does not require mixing. A chemically cured resin (autocuring resin) has two components which are gently mixed together to avoid incorporating air bubbles.

9.2.7 Sealant application

A small disposable brush or applicator, supplied by the manufacturer, is used to apply the sealant. The sealant is applied to the pits and fissures and up the etched cuspal slopes. If a light-cured material has been choosen, the light should be placed directly over the sealant, but should not touch it. The sealant is exposed for the full time recommended by the manufacturer to cure it. It is essential to time this carefully, as an incompletely cured material is doomed to failure. In addition, with a molar tooth, the light source should be directed at the distal part of the occlusal surface for the curing time and then moved to the mesial aspect for a similar time. Any buccal or palatal groove or pit should be similarly cured with the light source directly over it.

Most chemically cured sealants polymerize in 1–3 minutes and the manufacturer's instructions should be consulted to check the setting time of the particular material chosen.

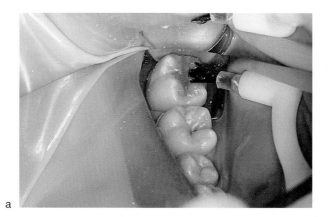

a

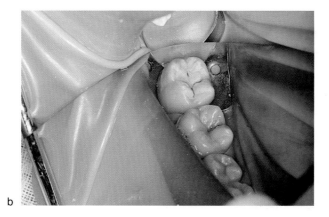

b

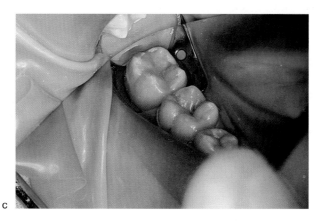

c

Figure 9.8. (a) Application of the etchant gel to the occlusal surfce of a lower second molar. (b) The dried etched area appears matt and white. (c) The completed fissure sealant. Note it has been applied within the etched area to ensure marginal seal. (By courtesy of Professor G. Roberts.)

The outer surface layer of any sealant will not polymerize, due to the inhibiting effect of oxygen in the atmosphere. Thus the sealant will always appear to have a greasy film after polymerization (Figure 9.8c).

9.2.8 Checking the occlusion

The rubber dam is now removed and the occlusion checked with articulating paper. It is considered acceptable to allow any high spots to be abraded away when unfilled fissure sealants are used, but with filled materials it is wiser to reduce high spots by grinding with a small round diamond stone in a conventional handpiece.

9.2.9 Recall and reassessment

It cannot be stressed too strongly that a fissure-sealed tooth is not immune from caries. A well-bonded sealant will prevent decay, but a leaking sealant is a recipe for disaster. For this reason, fissure-sealed teeth must be reviewed with the same care as unfilled or restored surfaces. This means that at every recall visit the teeth must be isolated with cotton-wool rolls and dried. The sealant is then checked visually. Any discoloration of the sealant, the margin of the sealant, or the underlying enamel must be viewed with suspicion as this may indicate leakage. A careful check should be made for partial or complete loss of the material. Coloured and filled resins are easier to see than the colourless and unfilled materials. However, the latter have the advantage that caries beneath them can be detected as a brown discoloration. In addition to a visual check, some operators advocate the use of a Briault probe to check that the sealant is firmly attached to the tooth and cannot be lifted off. Finally, at appropriate recall intervals, bitewing radiographs of sealed teeth must be carefully checked for signs of caries. Operative intervention is called for if caries in dentine is seen.

A sealant which is partly lost (Figure 9.9) or one where a margin is discoloured can be repaired by removing as much of the old sealant as possible, re-etching, and applying fresh sealant. Provided a clean surface is produced, new sealant will bond to the old material although this bond is not as strong as the original intact material.

9.2.10 The cost–effectiveness of sealants

Some attempts have been made to assess the cost-effectiveness of sealants. If every tooth with an occlusal surface were to be fissure sealed, fissure sealing would become more expensive than the alternative approach, which is the restoration of carious teeth. However, this 'blunderbuss' approach would not be a correct use for sealants because not all teeth are going to decay. Thus prescription of sealants must be based on an assessment of caries risk, which is best judged by past and present caries activity.

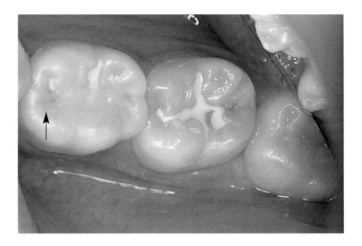

Figure 9.9. Part of the sealant has been lost and it should be repaired.

If fissure sealants were only to be used on first permanent molars, soon after eruption of these teeth, the procedure would probably be cost-effective. However, if caries risk is correctly assessed, not all those teeth will need to be fissure sealed. In a population with a falling caries rate, preventive efforts in the dental practice must be targeted at those most in need.

In addition, the value of a successful sealant must not be costed in terms of clinical time and materials alone. The technique is atraumatic, in contrast to operative dentistry. On the other hand, research has shown that placing a restoration in a tooth can start a restorative cycle where restorations tend to be removed and replaced every 5–10 years with a consequent increase in size of the cavity. Eventually the tooth structure is so weakened that a crown is required, and a failed crown may lead to extraction.

9.3 CARIES REMOVAL[6]

This section is going to be contentious! The current operative tradition is:
- Remove necrotic carious dentine and infected tissue with an excavator or slowly rotating round bur until hard dentine is reached.
- Now remove sufficent tooth structure to obtain a cavity suitable for the filling material of choice.
- Protect the pulpo-dential complex from further damage by placing a restoration that seals the cavity. It appears important to prevent penetration of microorganisms. Research seems to show that it is this bacterial ingress that potentially damages the pulp, rather than any toxological effect of the dental material.

However, this concept does not really fit with present knowledge of the carious process which occurs in the biofilm. It is the interaction of this biofilm with the dental tissues that results in the carious lesion.

The nub of the question is this: in the advanced dentine lesion, what is driving the carious process? Is it the bacteria in the biofilm or the bacteria in the infected dentine, or both? Logic would suggest that if the process is in the biofilm and the reflection is in the lesion, then all that must be removed is the biofilm and the lesion will arrest. There is support for this concept when the active root caries lesion is considered. The dentine is infected, but this infected dentine does not have to be removed by the dentist to arrest the process. With regular plaque removal and fluoride application an active root surface lesion gradually changes, with its surface becoming shiny, smooth, and hard on probing[7]. Over a period of months the heavily infected soft surface is gradually worn away and the lesion becomes shiny and hard.

Well, this argument may be acceptable with an accessible root surface lesion, but what about the cavitated lesion? Is it possible just to put a lid on the infected, demineralized dentine, sealing it from the oral environment? Are there dangers in leaving this infected tissue? What happens to the entombed microorganisms? Conversely, are there dangers to the pulp in complete and vigorous excavation?

9.3.1 Placing fissure sealants over carious dentine[6]

When sealants are placed over carious dentine, lesions apparently arrest both clinically and radiographically. Investigations of the fate of the sealed bacteria show a decrease in microorganisms with time or their complete elimination provided the sealants remain in place.

9.3.2 Stepwise excavation[6]

Stepwise excavation is a technique where only part of the soft dentine caries is removed at the first visit during the active phase of caries progression. The cavity is restored and re-opened after a period of weeks for further excavation before definitive restoration. The idea is to arrest progression of the lesion and allow formation of tertiary dentine to make pulpal exposure less likely.

There are at least a dozen studies of stepwise excavation and they vary in the amount of carious dentine removed at the first excavation, the restorative material used and the time to re-entry. However, irrespective of these variations, the clinical success is high; exposure is usually avoided; the dentine is altered on re-entry being dryer, harder, and darker. There are substantial reductions in the number of microorganisms that can be cultivated on re-entry. Intriguingly, there is some evidence that the surviving organisms are no longer representative of a cariogenic flora. This might indicate that the organisms within the infected dentine have been starved of nutrients by the restoration and the reparative processes of tubular sclerosis and tertiary dentine formation.

In addition to all these studies, there are two randomized controlled clinical trials where stepwise excavation is compared to conventional caries removal. Both these studies strongly support the stepwise approach in order to avoid pulp exposure.

9.3.3 Why re-enter?

In the 1960s your author, then a dental student, was told about stepwise excavation. The teacher (Professor Pickard of Manual fame[8]) was a keen gardener as well as a dentist and likened re-entry to 'digging up bulbs to see if they were growing!'. There is now a clinical study giving 10-year results of fillings placed in occlusal lesions where soft, demineralized dentine was left and acid-etched composite restorations placed.[9] There were control groups with conventional caries removal and restoration. The experimental restorations, where the infected dentine was left, remained clinically satisfactory. There was no pulpitis, no pulp death. The lesions must have arrested. The infected dentine could not have been driving the carious process, once the cavity was sealed.

This leaves our current operative tradition up the biological creek without a paddle! There is no evidence it is deleterious to leave infected dentine before sealing the cavity. Indeed, this cautious approach may be preferable to vigorous excavation because fewer pulps will be exposed and sealing the dentine from the oral environment encourages the arrest of lesion progression. The reparative processes of tubular sclerosis and tertiary dentine are encouraged, thus reducing the permeability of the remaining dentine. The residual microorganisms are now in a very different environment. They are entombed by the seal of the restoration on one side and the reduced permeability of the remaining dentine on the other. The apparent irrelevance of the infected dentine is biologically logical if it is accepted that the carious process occurs in the biofilm and its reflection is the lesion in the dental hard tissues.

9.3.4 Caries removal in the clinic

The above has been a most contentious discussion. Read the literature and discuss with your teachers. These arguments will have a strong bearing on the future of restorative dentistry. Well-controlled clinical studies need to be conducted, in combination with various laboratory and microbiological studies, in order to understand more and explain these intriguing observations.

In the meantime the author would suggest the following approach in the clinic:

- When removing caries make the enamel–dentine junction hard but do not worry about stain unless there is an appearance problem, e.g. in an anterior tooth. Staining is irrelevent to bacterial recovery.
- Excavate demineralized dentine over the pulpal surface to the level of firm dentine provided there is no liklihood of pulpal exposure.
- Deep lesions, in symptomless vital teeth, should be gently excavated. Soft, demineralized dentine may remain where its removal might expose the pulp. A permanent restoration is placed. Do not re-enter.
- Where it is not possible to remove soft, infected dentine (perhaps the patient is anxious or not cooperative), seal in the infected dentine. In a symptomless, vital tooth, this should have a high success rate.

9.4 STABLIZATION OF ACTIVE DISEASE WITH TEMPORARY DRESSINGS

When a patient presents with multiple carious lesions, a combined preventive and operative approach will be required. This approach must include a careful history and examination, diagnosis of the cause of the disease, extraction of teeth which are obviously unsavable, institution of preventive measures, and stabilization of large, active lesions. All lesions where pulpal involvement looks likely on a radiograph should be treated in the following way.

- The tooth should initially be tested to determine whether the pulp is vital. If it is, a local anaesthetic is given and access gained to the carious dentine, and demineralized tissue removed as described in the previous section. A glass ionomer cement temporary dressing is placed.
- Where caries has resulted in frank exposure of a vital pulp, removal of the pulp is often advisable to prevent pain. Eventually such teeth require root canal therapy if they are to be saved, but initially the pulp cavity may be dressed with a mild antiseptic on cotton wool and the tooth restored with a glass ionomer cement as a temporary filling. Where inadequate anaesthesia or insufficient time preclude complete removal of the coronal and radicular pulp, a vital exposure can be dressed with a corticosteroid antibiotic preparation before placing a temporary filling. These products are unrivalled in their ability to suppress the inflammatory process and hence the pain of pulpitis, but root canal therapy is the eventual treatment of choice if the tooth is to be saved.
- Where grossly carious teeth are found to be non-vital, but the teeth are restorable, the pulp cavity may be dressed with a mild antiseptic on cotton wool and the tooth restored temporarily. If, however, the patient has symptoms of acute apical infection, thorough debridement of

the root canal system is required before placement of a mild antiseptic dressing in the coronal pulp chamber and temporary restoration of the tooth.

Stabilization of active, advanced lesions in this way is an essential part of deciding the eventual treatment plan for the patient. It may be that some of these teeth are found to be unrestorable and their extraction will therefore be advised. It is only after such careful investigation that the dentist can estimate the extent of restorative treatment required, such as the number of root fillings. Stabilization makes plaque control in these areas possible and ensures that toothache is not experienced in one tooth while many restorative hours are devoted to another.

In addition, during these stabilization appointments, dentist and patient will be getting to know one another. Preventive measures can be instituted and the dentist can begin to gauge the patient's attitude towards disease control in their own mouth. If cooperation with dietary and plaque control seems to be forthcoming, a treatment plan that preserves as many teeth as possible will be justified. If, on the other hand, the patient appears uninterested and disinclined to play their essential role in disease control, a treatment involving some extractions and simple restorations may have more chance of success in the long run.

Definitive restorations should not be started in such a patient until prevention has been instituted and grossly carious teeth stabilized.

Further reading and references

1. Elderton, R. J. and Mjör, I. A. (1988) Treatment planning. In: Hörsted-Bindsler, P. and Mjör, I. A. (eds) *Modern concepts in operative dentistry*. Munksgaard, Copenhagen.
2. Fejerskov, O. and Kidd, E. A. M. (eds) (2003) *Dental caries*. Ch.15: The role of operative treatment. Blackwell Munksgaard, Oxford.
3. Carvalho, J. C., Thylstrup, A., and Ekstrand, K. (1992) Results after 3 years non-operative occlusal caries treatment of erupting permanent first molars. *Commun. Dent. Oral Epidemiol.*, **20**, 187–192.
4. British Society of Paediatric Dentistry (2000) Fissure sealants in paediatric dentistry, a policy document. *Int. J. Paed. Dent.*, **10**, 174–177.
5. Locker, D. and Jokovic, A. (2003) The use of pit and fissure sealants in preventing caries in the permanent dentition of children. *Br. Dent. J.*, **195**, 375–378.
6. Kidd, E. A. M. (2004) How 'clean' must a cavity be before restoration? *Caries Res.*, **38**, 305–313.
7. Nyvad, B. and Fejerskov, O. (1986) Active root-caries converted into inactive caries as a response to oral hygiene. *Scand. J. Dent. Res.*, **94**, 281–284.
8. Kidd, E. A. M., Smith, B. G. N., and Watson, T. F. (2003) *Pickard's manual of operative dentistry*, 8th edn. Oxford University Press, Oxford.
9. Mertz-Fairhurst, E., Curtis, J. W., Ergle, J. W., and Rueggeberg, F. A. (1998) Ultra-conservative and cariostatic sealed restorations: results at year 10. *J. Am. Dent. Assoc.*, **129**, 55–66.

Index

acesulfame-K 102
Actinomyces spp. 3
active carious lesions 2, 8, 36
animal experiments 91
approximal surface caries, diagnosis 50–5
 bitewing radiography 51–3
 clinical-visual examination 50
 tactile examination 51
 tooth separation 54–5
 transmitted light 53–4
arrested (inactive) carious lesion 8, 9,
 26–8, 36–7
aspartame 102

bacteria
 acidogenic 4
 aciduric 4
 microcolonies 3
 pathogenic properties 4
biofilm 2
bitewing radiographs 44–5
 approximal surface caries 51–3
 recurrent caries 59
body language 145–7
bottle caries 11
breast feeding 94

carbohydrate, and caries formation 7–8
caries 2
 classification of 8–11
 diagnosis 41–65
 site of 4–6
caries activity 12, 65
caries removal 171–4
 see also fissure sealing
caries risk 60
 assessment of 60–4
 dental history 62
 diet 62–3
 medical history 60–2
 oral hygiene 62
 risk groups 94

saliva 63–4
social and demographic factors 64
carious exposure 33
carious lesions 3, 5, 41
 active 2, 8, 36
 arrested (inactive) 8, 9, 26–8, 36–7
carious process 3
cavitation 31
 dentine changes 32–3
chewing gum 84
children 15–17
 chronically sick 105
 toothpaste use 82
 young 105
chlorhexidine 82–5
 control of caries 85
 gel 139–40
 long-term effects 85
 mechanism of action, dosage, and
  delivery 83–4
 side effects
  desquamation of oral mucosa 84–5
  parotid gland swelling 84
  staining 84
  taste 84
communication *see* patient communication

dead tracts 32
def index 12–13
demineralization 2, 31, 32, 111–12
dental floss 74–5, 76
dental history 62
dentine 30–1
 cavitation 32–3
 reparative 33
 structure 22
 tertiary 30
dentine caries 32–3
 active 36–7
 arrested 36–7
 colour of 39
 microbiology 36
 tubular sclerosis 30
DEPCAT status 17
DIAGNOdent 49

hydroxyapatite 22
hyposalivation 63

incidence 12
intense sweeteners 102
interdental brushes 75–7
interdental cleaning 74–7
intrinsic sugars 93
isomalt 103

laser fluorescence 49–50
levels of disease 43–4
liquefaction foci 32
locus of control 142, 156–7

Maillard reaction 39
mannitol 102
medical history 60–2
microbial succession 4
microcolonies 3
mirrors 71
modification of carious process 18–19
mottled enamel 110

non-milk extrinsic sugars 93
non-specific plaque hypothesis 4
nursing caries 11
nutritive sweeteners 102–3

occlusal caries 5
operative treatment 19, 159–75
  caries removal 171–4
  definition of 160–1
  fissure sealing 163–71
  reasons for 161–2
  temporary dressings 174–5
  timing of 162–3
oral hygiene 18, 62

patient advice 81–2, 148–50
  amount of information 148–9
  involvement of patient 148
  non-verbal communication 143,
    145–7
  telephone reminders 150
  timing of 149–50
  use of other senses 148
patient behaviour change 155
patient communication 143–7
  bodily contact 146–7
  bodily posture 146
  clothes and appearance 147
  distortion 145
  eye contact 145–6
  facial expression 145
  forgetting 144–5
  gestures and bodily movements 146
  jargon 144
  listening and empathy 144
  open and closed questions 143–4
  spatial behaviour 147
  tone of voice 145
patient compliance 143
  care 152
  diagnosis of problem 150
  enthusiasm 151
  factors affecting 142
  failure of 156–7
  negotiation 152–3
  patient's beliefs 151
  praise 152
  realistic goals 153
  reinforcement and follow-up 154,
    156
  relevance of advice 151
  scoring 154
  trust 152
patients' role 142–3
pellicle 3
pit and fissure caries, diagnosis 47–50
  clinical-visual and radiographic
    examination 47–9
  laser fluorescence 49–50
plaque 3–7
  acid production in 88
  pH 7
plaque control 67–85, 139
  advice to patients 81–2
  chlorhexidine 82–5
  interdental cleaning 74–7
  professional 80–1
  toothbrushing 72–4
  toothpastes 77–80
pregnant and nursing mothers
  104–5
prevalence 12, 14–15
primary caries 8